PANOS DOSSIER

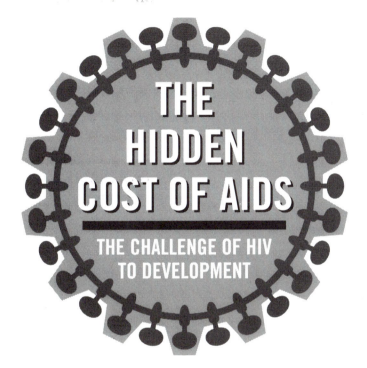

THE HIDDEN COST OF AIDS

THE CHALLENGE OF HIV TO DEVELOPMENT

T   ...   UTE

LON   ...   NGTON

ACKNOWLEDGEMENTS

Panos wishes to acknowledge the help given by many individuals and organisations across the world in compiling this dossier. Many people credited in the text also gave valuable background information or reviewed the draft text. Space does not allow us to thank everyone by name, but we would like to include the following: Martha Ainsworth, Maxine Ankrah, Mike Bailey, Tony Barnett, Patrick Brenny, Rodolfo Bulatao, Simon Burne, Charles Cameron, Ian Campbell, Michel Carael, James Deane, Monica Dolan, Don Edwards, Steven Forsythe, Susan Foster, Geoff Garnett, Bob Grose, Pamela Hartigan, Barbara Heinzen, Sue Lucas, Claudia Garcia Moreno, Daniel Nelson, Elizabeth Ngugi, David Norse, Maura O'Donohue, Mead Over, Jane Rowley, Peer Sieben, Alan Whiteside, and individuals at the following organisations: Brazilian Inter-disciplinary AIDS Association, ACORD, Care, Concern, Global AIDS Policy Coalition, Save the Children Fund, World Bank, WHO and World Vision.

Published by Panos Publications Ltd
9 White Lion Street
London N1 9PD, UK
British Library Cataloguing in Publication Data
Hidden Cost of AIDS: challenge of HIV to development
I. Series
616.97
ISBN 1-870670-29-9

Funding for *The Hidden Cost of AIDS* was provided by the Ministry of Foreign Affairs, Denmark, Swiss Development Cooperation (DDA), CAFOD and Redd Barna (Save the Children, Norway). The Panos AIDS and Development Unit also receives financial support from the Swedish International Development Authority and the Ford Foundation. It provides independent accessible information on the development implications of HIV/AIDS and works with others, particularly in the developing world, to increase their capacity to report on the disease.

Any judgements expressed in this document should not be taken to represent the views of any funding agency. Signed articles do not necessarily reflect the views of Panos or any of its funding agencies. Except where specifically stated, it is not suggested that any individual referred to or pictured in this dossier has contracted HIV.

Research on this dossier was undertaken by Martin Foreman and Fiona Belton. It was written by Martin Foreman and Olivia Bennett, with Michele Karam. Other writers are acknowledged where their contribution appears in the text.

The Panos Institute is an information and policy studies institute, dedicated to working in partnership with others towards greater public understanding of sustainable development. Panos has offices in London, Paris and Washington DC. For more information about Panos contact Juliet Heller, Panos London.

Managing editor: Olivia Bennett
Production: Sally O'Leary
Picture research: Adrian Evans Illustrations: Philip Davies
Cover design: The Graphic Partnership
Printed in Great Britain by The Bath Press, Bath

Contents

Introduction

In March 1987, the Panos Institute held a meeting in Talloires, France, bringing together leaders of development assistance agencies with the object of persuading them to take HIV/AIDS more seriously [1]. When they arrived, most of them saw HIV/AIDS as just another health problem: a headline-grabbing disease which seemed to be spreading fast in parts of Africa and the Caribbean. By the time they left, most were convinced that HIV/AIDS had the potential to threaten many of the achievements of Third World development.

Five years after Talloires, HIV/AIDS is beginning to fulfil that potential. Once again, there is an urgent need to focus attention on the development aspects of the disease, rather than on the more narrow health issues.

But why all the fuss about HIV/AIDS? After all, it only kills about 100,000 people a year worldwide. That's fairly small compared with 1 million a year from malaria, 3 million from tuberculosis, 4 million from diarrhoeal disease, 5 million from cancer, and about 12 million from heart and other cardiovascular diseases [2]. Why should HIV/AIDS be seen as such a threat?

There are a number of reasons, and the first is the peculiar nature of HIV, the virus which causes AIDS. HIV is mainly transmitted in sexual intercourse. Since few human societies talk openly and honestly about sex, this makes HIV/AIDS difficult to discuss; and since sex is a very private activity, it makes the transmission of HIV difficult to control.

HIV itself doesn't cause any illness at all. Instead, it steadily lowers the body's resistance to other disease organisms, and it is these other infections which cause sickness and death. Many cases of AIDS are officially reported as being pneumonia, or TB, or diarrhoea—rather as if someone hit by a car was said to have died from bleeding or concussion.

Medical science has so far proved singularly ineffective in defending us against HIV. There is no vaccine to protect against infection; and no treatments which can cure those who are infected, although some very expensive drugs can, at the price of many side effects, slow down the progress of illness. And once AIDS develops, it seems invariably to be fatal.

The second reason why HIV/AIDS is taken so seriously is its extraordinary capacity for growth. In 1992, about 100,000 people probably died of AIDS all over the world; by the end of the century the figure is expected to be at least 400,000 a year. Malaria, TB, heart disease, cancer: no other disease is growing, or is likely to grow, at anything like this speed. And in spite of HIV/AIDS campaigns in many countries, there is little evidence so far of any slowdown in the spread of the epidemic. By the end of the century, at least 40 million people —and perhaps as many as 100 million—are expected to have been infected by HIV.

The third reason why HIV/AIDS is taken so seriously is the long incubation period between infection and illness. On average, it takes about 10 years for someone infected with HIV to develop AIDS. During incubation, she or he will show few if any symptoms, but will be able to infect other people.

This long incubation period is rare in human disease, and it means that changes in HIV transmission rates take 10 years to show results. Such a long gap between cause and effect makes it extraordinarily difficult to persuade individuals or governments to take the pandemic seriously. People dying today represent those infected 10 years ago: the results of anything we do now to reduce transmission will not be apparent until the next century.

The fourth reason why HIV/AIDS is more serious than many numerically more common diseases is because of whom it attacks. Some diseases—measles and diarrhoea, for example —hit mainly infants and children; others, such as heart disease and cancer, affect mainly the old. But because HIV is predominantly transmitted sexually, AIDS mainly kills people in their 20s, 30s and 40s. A major increase in deaths among these age groups, the most productive section of society, will have much greater social and economic effects than deaths among children or old people.

In the Third World in particular, it has become increasingly clear over the past five years that HIV/AIDS challenges many of the assumptions upon which development is based. Nearly every sector of a nation's economy will be affected—in ways that are not yet always predictable or obvious.

This dossier seeks to cast some light on what the impacts of HIV/AIDS will be, on ways in which they can be reduced, and on how we can prepare for those impacts which are inevitable.

The cost to development

One of the success stories of the past four decades has been the reduction in disease in even the poorest countries. The pandemic not only threatens to stop that progress, but to throw it into reverse. Life expectancy in some countries may start to fall.

Most epidemics, from influenza to the Black Death, kill mainly the weakest, and especially the very young and the old. HIV is no respecter of the survival of the fittest. In fact, because HIV hits active young adults the hardest, it could be described as the killer of the fittest. The population it leaves behind is less able to cope, because it has lost its most productive sector.

Education is both a cornerstone of development and a measure of its success. Especially in the early stages of an epidemic, HIV/AIDS tends to affect disproportionately the more skilled and the better educated. So the cost of even maintaining existing numbers of nurses or engineers, for example, starts to rise. As an HIV/AIDS epidemic grows, it tends to focus more on the poorest and the most disadvantaged. Again, education suffers, as children are kept away from school to care for sick relatives, or the family can no longer afford to send them to school.

Any community needs self-confidence to undertake development. HIV/AIDS can undermine that process, through the despair and poverty that a severe epidemic can bring. At the same time, already poor communities are often too concerned about immediate needs to give any serious consideration to a disease whose impacts lie hidden 10 years in the future. In rural areas of the Third World, as rates of infection rise, food production is likely to drop. Nutrition levels will probably fall, and food supplies to the cities may decline. Cash crop production may be affected, reducing governments' ability to finance food imports. Industry is likely to suffer too. Labour costs may rise as shortages develop, and employers may face spiralling medical costs as well as the expense of training new people to replace those who die.

The evidence in this dossier suggests that HIV/AIDS will have a more complex set of impacts than had previously been imagined. The picture is incomplete, and still relies too heavily on studies from Central and East Africa, although if little is done to contain the epidemic the impacts may be as severe elsewhere.

To some, this picture may be depressing and demotivating. Such a reaction would be foolish and short-sighted. There are at least three important reasons why a better understanding of the development impacts of HIV/AIDS is positive and valuable.

The first is that a measure of the true costs of a severe

HIV/AIDS epidemic provides the strongest argument for trying to prevent one happening. Medical science has not yet given us the tools to stop the spread of HIV, but we know how to slow it down—predominantly through changes in sexual behaviour. The cash benefits of action against HIV/AIDS are immense. One calculation, for example, suggests that $100 million spent in anti-HIV/AIDS activities in Thailand in 1991-92 could eventually result in 3.5 million fewer people being infected, and in $5.1 billion being saved. Spending $1 now to save $51 later does sound quite a good investment [3].

The second argument for taking a realistic look at the likely impacts of HIV/AIDS is so we can take development as well as health measures to undermine the factors which facilitate its spread. We can try to emphasise rural development and reduce drift to the cities; to strengthen a community's mutual support mechanisms; to ensure that health education tackles head-on the delicate issues around sexually transmitted diseases; to reduce the poverty and inequality on which the virus thrives; to reduce the lack of power many women have over their own sex lives, so they have a real choice between safe and unsafe sex.

There is a third reason why we must have the courage to look at the likely impacts of the pandemic. If we know the probable impacts of HIV/AIDS, we can take steps to mitigate or to live with its consequences.

We can design agricultural policies to take account of the loss of time and labour with which farmers will be coping, perhaps by switching to less labour-intensive varieties of crops. We can prepare economic policies which recognise the potential changes to the age-structure of the labour force. We can plan for the social upheaval and especially the effect on children, many of whom may be orphaned, and adjust schooling systems to allow for the time off which some children may need to care for dying parents.

Thinking about the likely development impacts of HIV/AIDS is not going to make them go away. But it should enable us to improve the way we handle those impacts.

HIV/AIDS carries a high price, and one that has so far been largely hidden. This dossier is designed to bring the hidden costs of HIV/AIDS into the open. There are ways of reducing these costs, if we act in time. And if we know the size of the price-tag in advance, we may be able to find easier ways of paying for it.

Jon Tinker
President, Panos Institute

CHAPTER 1

The HIV pandemic

The rapid spread of the Human Immunodeficiency Virus (HIV) across the globe in the past decade is inextricably linked to the poverty and powerlessness in which the majority of the world's population lives. With non-sterile needles and contaminated blood playing a minor role, the spread of HIV is predominantly driven by sexual intercourse. The widespread existence of untreated sexually transmitted diseases (STDs) facilitates the transmission of HIV and may hasten the development of Acquired Immune Deficiency Syndrome (AIDS). Frequent sexual partner change—which for many women is a reflection of low economic and social status rather than of choice—increases the risk of contracting the virus. The countries hardest hit, most of which are in the developing world, have the fewest resources to deal with the effects of HIV/AIDS or to contain its spread.

What is being measured?
The commonest means of measuring the pandemic has been to add up the number of AIDS cases reported by ministries of health to the World Health Organization (WHO). However, this method is misleading, partly because the figures are cumulative and include not only those who are currently ill but all who have died of AIDS since the disease was first identified [1], and partly because not all AIDS cases are reported. This is due to the fact that not all people with AIDS are seen by doctors, doctors sometimes fail to diagnose the disease, and the administrative and financial means are not always available to record all diagnosed cases. WHO therefore estimates that worldwide 1.7 million adults had developed or died from AIDS by July 1992, rather than the 500,000 officially reported [2].

Even if these factors are taken into account, a description of the pandemic restricted to the number of AIDS cases is misleading. By concentrating on those who have fallen ill, it ignores those who are infected but who have not yet developed symptoms definable as AIDS. Worldwide, perhaps 10 times as

HIV and AIDS

AIDS (Acquired Immune Deficiency Syndrome) is the name given to the fatal clinical condition that results from long-term infection with HIV (Human Immunodeficiency Virus) [36]. HIV progressively damages the body's immune defence system, preventing the body from protecting itself against infections that it would otherwise render harmless. These opportunistic infections include tuberculosis, Kaposi's sarcoma (a tumour primarily affecting the skin), *Pneumocystis carinii* (a form of pneumonia), diarrhoea and severe weight loss. Over time HIV weakens the immune system to the extent that several opportunistic infections are present at once; death is not caused directly by HIV but by one or more of these infections.

HIV does not appear to increase vulnerability to every disease. It may affect the rapidity with which syphilis develops [37], but there does not appear to be a similarly close link between HIV/AIDS and other endemic diseases such as malaria, meningococcal disease and sleeping sickness [38].

Because a variety of infections can occur in a person with HIV prior to a diagnosis of AIDS, some experts prefer to talk about "HIV disease" rather than HIV infection and AIDS. WHO has proposed a four part staging system to describe the patterns of ill health resulting from HIV infection. AIDS (the fourth stage) is diagnosed when the combination of symptoms meets the appropriate WHO definition of the syndrome [39]. Slightly different definitions of AIDS are used in Africa, Latin America and North America to meet regional variations in opportunistic infections and diagnostic capabilities.

Almost 100% of those who contract HIV develop AIDS. The period between becoming infected and developing AIDS averages 10 years in adults. Infants born with HIV may progress rapidly to AIDS, developing symptoms after four months, or may not develop AIDS for several years [40]. Availability of treatment and other factors mean that even with treatment, average adult life expectancy after diagnosis of AIDS ranges from six to 12 months in the developing world and one to two years in the industrialised world.

Being infected with HIV does not automatically mean that a person has AIDS or is ill. With or without symptoms of AIDS, a person with HIV (also known as a person who is HIV-positive or seropositive) is permanently infected and permanently infectious to others through the means of transmission described opposite.

many people are HIV-positive as have AIDS, a ratio that rises to over 100 in South and Southeast Asia as a result of more recent spread of the virus. Each person with HIV is permanently infected, may infect others and is almost certain to develop symptoms and eventually die. Because of the time lapse between contracting HIV and falling ill with AIDS—an average of 10 years—a definition of the pandemic restricted to AIDS is no more than a record of the past and gives little idea of the extent of the problem today. That can be determined only by estimating the number of people currently infected.

The Global Picture

Authorities agree, therefore, that the true pandemic is one of HIV, not AIDS. It is estimated that, worldwide, up to 12 million adults (over 6 million men and 5 million women) are infected with HIV. This represents 1 in 250 of the world's adult population. One million children had contracted HIV by early 1992. Over 80% of all these cases were in the developing world [3], with infection rates reaching more than 1 in 10 adults in some communities. Because sexual intercourse is the major route of HIV transmission, the vast majority of those infected are between 15 and 44 years of age. Because of mother-to-child transmission, the number of women infected has major implications for the number of children likely to be born HIV-positive. There are currently wide regional differences in the proportions of population infected and in the ratio of men to women infected (see map).

Heterosexual intercourse accounted for 70%-75% of all

HIV transmission

HIV is transmitted in semen, vaginal fluid and blood. Transmission of HIV can occur only in the following ways:

* through unprotected (without use of a condom) vaginal or anal intercourse with an infected person. A few cases of HIV transmission have been attributed to oral intercourse;
* through infected blood—in transfusion, blood products, the use of contaminated needles, syringes or other skin-piercing instruments in injecting drug use, medical and quasi-medical use;
* from an infected mother to her child before or during birth; the risk of transmitting infection is estimated at 30%. Recent evidence suggests that most transmission takes place during delivery [41]. There is evidence that breast-feeding is also a route of HIV transmission [42], but WHO recommends that "where infectious diseases and malnutrition are the main cause of infant deaths and the infant mortality rate is high, breast-feeding should be the usual advice to pregnant women, including those who are HIV-infected [43]."

HIV does not survive easily outside the body. It is not transmitted in the everyday circumstances of home, school, workplace, restaurants or any public place, on toilet seats, by hugging, kissing or shaking hands, sharing eating or drinking utensils, by coughing or by mosquito or other insect bites.

HIV-1 and HIV-2

The term HIV refers to two similar viruses: HIV-1 and HIV-2. Both viruses reproduce by using the genetic materials of the cells they invade and both gradually disable the body's immune system. HIV-2, however, is less virulent than HIV-1 [44].

HIV-1 is found throughout the world. HIV-2 is prevalent in West Africa, although it has been detected in other parts of the continent and some countries in the Americas, Europe and Asia. In recent years HIV-1 seems to be spreading faster in West Africa than HIV-2.

SUMMARY *Summary* *Summary*

infections worldwide by 1992. Other means of transmission were estimated as: male homosexual intercourse 5%-10%; blood transfusion 3%-5%; injecting drug use 5%-10%; mother-to-child 5%-10% [4]. These are not static figures. The proportion of cases resulting from heterosexual transmission continues to rise while the proportion due to transmission through contaminated blood or blood products continues to fall.

Patterns of infection

Although heterosexual intercourse is the principal means of transmission worldwide, the history of the epidemic has led to regional variations. In the industrialised countries of Australasia, North America and Western Europe, HIV/AIDS predominantly affects men who have sex with men, and injecting drug users. The rate of infection resulting from homosexual transmission has decreased significantly since the early 1980s, while heterosexual

Vaccines and treatments

Vaccines work by using fragments of the dead virus, or a weakened non-lethal version of the live virus, to stimulate the body's immune system. A number of technical problems are involved in developing a vaccine against HIV, including identifying the most appropriate strain of the virus and the best fragment to stimulate the immune system. A successful vaccine against HIV is not expected before the end of the century.

There are concerns over who is or should be controlling the development of, and determining the priority given to, vaccines and treatments: WHO, pharmaceutical companies, or governments. It is not clear to what extent developing country scientists and AIDS experts will participate in equal partnership with researchers from the North in designing and implementing vaccine trials. Developing country scientists are also voicing their disquiet over future trials and questioning the assumption that such trials should take place in the South. The present inequality of treatments for HIV/AIDS fuels concern in the developing world that even if their citizens take part in experimental vaccine trials they will be priced out of any future vaccines, which are likely to be prohibitively expensive.

Three types of treatment exist for people with AIDS:

* palliative care to reduce pain or discomfort caused by opportunistic infections;
* drugs to attack opportunistic infections;
* anti-viral drugs such as zidovudine (AZT) and ddI (didanosine) which attack HIV directly.

Treatment may alleviate symptoms and return a patient to temporary health, but even the most comprehensive treatment, including anti-viral drugs, cannot eradicate HIV and cure AIDS. There is some evidence that taking zidovudine before symptoms appear delays development of AIDS [45]. In most countries of the developing world, cost rules out the use of anti-viral drugs—the average annual cost of zidovudine is $1,200 and of ddI $2,000—while drugs to counter opportunistic infections are often available only in large city hospitals.

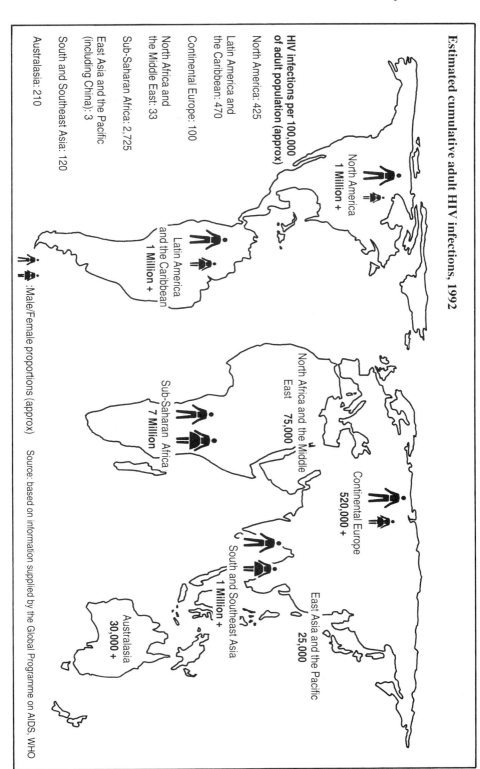

Estimated cumulative adult HIV infections, 1992

HIV infections per 100,000 of adult population (approx)

North America: 425

Latin America and the Caribbean: 470

Continental Europe: 100

North Africa and the Middle East: 33

Sub-Saharan Africa: 2,725

East Asia and the Pacific (including China): 3

South and Southeast Asia: 120

Australasia: 210

:Male/Female proportions (approx)

Source: based on information supplied by the Global Programme on AIDS, WHO

North America 1 Million +

Latin America and the Caribbean 1 Million +

North Africa and the Middle East 75,000

Sub-Saharan Africa 7 Million

Continental Europe 520,000 +

South and Southeast Asia 1 Million +

East Asia and the Pacific 25,000

Australasia 30,000 +

transmission is rising slowly [5].

In sub-Saharan Africa, heterosexual intercourse has been the principal mode of spread since the epidemic was first detected, and accounts for over 80% of infections. As with other sexually transmitted diseases, more women than men have contracted HIV; the male to female ratio is approximately 1:1.2. At least three-quarters of a million infants are estimated to have been born with HIV by 1992.

In Latin America and the Caribbean, where one million people are believed to be infected, spread of HIV began among men who have sex with men, and injecting drug users. Since the 1980s, in many countries of the region sexual transmission between men and women has become a major, possibly predominant, mode of spread; as a result it is estimated that 10,000 children in the region have been born HIV-positive.

HIV is spreading rapidly in South and Southeast Asia, particularly in India and Thailand. Among injecting drug users infection has been detected at levels of 50% in Bangkok,

Sexual behaviour

Worldwide, ignorance surrounds a key factor in the spread of HIV—patterns of sexual intercourse and how they vary between and within communities. Only now is research under way in a number of countries into such questions as who has sex, their age, their socio-economic background, how often they have sex, the age and background of their partners, and what sexual acts are performed.

HIV/AIDS throws a spotlight that reveals that in every society sexual behaviour is more varied than cultural norms suggest. Homosexuality, prostitution and non-monogamous partnerships are universal; where they are strongly discouraged, the frequency may be reduced but the behaviour itself is seldom eliminated.

Not only social attitudes, but social conditions influence patterns of sexual behaviour. These may become a further factor facilitating transmission of HIV. There is, for example, evidence to suggest that in cities and communities where there is a high ratio of men to women, the incidence of infection rises rapidly in the community as a whole. In this situation, because relatively few women are sexually active, they have more partners and are more vulnerable to infection; thus in turn they are more likely to infect their partners. Such has been the pattern in Kigali, Rwanda, where there are 50% more men than women aged 20-39, and is the likely pattern in the urban slums of India, where there are also many more young men than women. Unless other factors (such as the incidence of STDs) play a major role, in communities where the sex ratio is more equal and therefore women have on average fewer partners, the incidence of infection rises more slowly [46].

Other factors facilitate or hinder HIV transmission in other communities, such as the pattern and prevalence of male bisexual behaviour in Latin America and elsewhere. Until such factors are better understood, however, detailed understanding of how the epidemic reached this point and how it may develop in future, will not be possible.

Thailand, and in the Indian state of Manipur, and 30% in Yangon, Myanmar (formerly Rangoon, Burma). Heterosexual transmission has resulted in an estimated 250,000 infections in the larger cities of India. In Thailand it is reported that nearly 70% of known new infections are in heterosexual men and women aged 15-29 [6].

Less information on HIV rates of infection is available from North Africa and the Middle East, but both heterosexual intercourse and injecting drug use have been implicated in transmission. Infection rates of 40% have been found among women prostitutes in one North African country and 14% in injecting drug users in one Gulf state.

In Central and Eastern Europe and the former USSR relatively few people—under 50,000—are believed to be infected. The groups predominantly affected vary from country to country and include homosexual and heterosexual men and injecting drug users. In the late 1980s, in Romania and parts of the former USSR, several hundred children and some mothers were infected by non-sterile needles in medical or quasi-medical settings.

A Series of Sub-epidemics

The pattern of HIV infection varies not only from continent to continent, but also within and between countries. Infection levels in the general population of the city of Kigali, Rwanda, for example, are five times higher than in Kinshasa in neighbouring Zaire (see Box opposite). In the Rakai district of Uganda, levels of infection vary widely, from a low of 1.2% in some areas to 52.8% in others [7]. Means of transmission also vary. In some Caribbean islands the epidemic is predominantly spread by injecting drug use and in others by heterosexual intercourse.

Such variations are better understood if HIV/AIDS is viewed as several sub-epidemics, affecting population groups differently as a result of associated social or physical factors. Sexual transmission accounts for most of these sub-epidemics, with local variations caused by contaminated blood and needles. Thus the situation in Thailand can be seen as consisting of one sub-epidemic among injecting drug users, another among women sex workers and their clients and a third among male sex workers and their clients. In Central Africa, HIV/AIDS affects upper-income men with a number of sexual partners and their usually monogamous wives, and lower-income men and women who frequently change sexual partners. In Brazil, one epidemic affects recipients of contaminated blood products and their partners, another affects injecting drug users, and a third homosexual and bisexual men and their partners.

India also provides evidence that HIV sub-epidemics can affect different social groups with little or no interaction between them, with its first sub-epidemic among poor women prostitutes in urban areas and their clients, and its second among drug-injecting middle- and upper-class youths in the northeastern states. Similarly, in the United States one sub-epidemic is among middle-class urban white males, who comprise the majority of infected gay (homosexual) men, and another is among poorer urban non-white men and women and is spread by drug injecting and by heterosexual intercourse.

However, most of these sub-epidemics overlap with others, while sexual intercourse transmits the virus to others who are not at "high risk" (see below). Analysing the factors that allow HIV to spread leads to greater understanding of the dynamics behind each of these sub-epidemics—and thus indicates the first steps that can be taken to slow down the pandemic.

Non-sexual Transmission

Contaminated syringes—syringes re-used without sterilisation —can transmit HIV and other diseases from one person to the next in drug injecting and medical or quasi-medical settings. The efficiency of transmission—close to 100% according to some experts [8]—explains the rapid spread of the virus where drug users or medical practitioners do not sterilise syringes.

Where conditions encourage sterilisation, transmission rates

People at risk

High-risk behaviour is sexual or drug-injecting behaviour which allows HIV to be transmitted from an infected person to an uninfected person. Any individual who practises such behaviour, however infrequently, is at risk of infection. Thus an individual may have only one sexual encounter, but if their partner has contracted HIV, they are at risk.

Some people's behaviour places them at repeated risk; for example, an injecting drug user may regularly share needles, or a person may have intercourse with several partners without using a condom. Such behaviour is not always from choice: a prostitute of either sex, for example, may not be able to insist that their client uses a condom. In epidemiological terms, these people form **high-risk groups**.

As this dossier demonstrates, high levels of preventable disease, low levels of education, inadequate health resources and a background of poverty, rapid urbanisation, social upheaval and marginalisation, all facilitate transmission of HIV. These conditions comprise **high-risk situations**, which are as great a factor in the spread of HIV/AIDS as individual behaviour [47].

are low. Rates of infection among injecting drug users in cities where clean syringes are easily available (for example, in Liverpool, UK, where it is less than 6%) are much lower than cities where clean syringes are difficult to obtain (for example, in New York, where it is 60%-70%) [9]. Hospital procedures in Western Europe mean that transmission in a medical setting is extremely rare. Unless instruments are sterilised, a risk of transmission remains in countries where injections are given by quasi-medical personnel and where male and female circumcision and scarification are carried out.

Men and women are at greater risk of infection if they have a history of other STDs

The efficiency of HIV transmission through transfusion of blood products is also close to 100% [10]. Where blood is not screened before transfusion, many people have been infected by this means; in parts of sub-Saharan Africa, where donors are often family members, it has been a factor in transmission from parents to children. Globally it is estimated that 3%-5% of HIV infections have been transmitted by blood and blood products.

Sexual Transmission

Sexual, specifically heterosexual, intercourse is the predominant mode of HIV transmission. Certain physical factors place both men and women at greater risk: the most significant of these are other STDs.

The role of STDs

Men and women are at greater risk of infection by HIV if they have a history of other STDs, particularly those associated with genital ulcerations such as chancroid, syphilis and genital herpes [11]. STDs which do not cause ulcers are also implicated [12].

Much of the rapid spread of HIV in the developing world can be attributed to high and rising rates of STDs, which are themselves spreading because of inadequate health services, which means most STDs remain untreated. The rate of infection among women, in particular, is difficult to document, since women with STDs often have few or no symptoms. In the 1970s, gonorrhoea and syphilis were 10-70 times higher in parts of Africa than in London [13]. Official estimates suggest there are 3 million new STD infections in India each year [14]. In parts of the industrialised world, after a period of long decline, the incidence of some STDs such as syphilis is rising. In 1990, with 250 million new infections occurring annually, WHO director-general Hiroshi Nakajima pointed out that "sexually transmitted infections and diseases have reached epidemic proportions globally [15]".

Other factors

Women are placed at greater risk by the fact that male-female transmission is more efficient than female-male: men are twice as likely to infect their female partners as vice versa [16].

It has been suggested that women are also placed at greater risk by:

- the use of intra-uterine contraceptive devices (IUDs) [17] and some traditional preparations applied before intercourse which may create inflammation [18];
- the effect of malnutrition, which results in greater likelihood of bruising the vagina during intercourse [19];
- intercourse before sexual maturity [20];
- the practice of female circumcision, although this has not been confirmed by epidemiological evidence [21].

Men are placed at greater risk of infection by:

- lack of circumcision; the foreskin traps vaginal fluid, provides a larger surface area for uptake of the virus and may be more susceptible to microscopic tears during sexual intercourse [22];
- intercourse during menstruation [23].

Other factors facilitating transmission of HIV include the following:

- the risk of acquiring HIV infection for the receiving partner in anal intercourse may be 10 times higher than in vaginal intercourse [24];
- individuals are more infectious for several months after contracting HIV and after the development of AIDS symptoms than at other times in the course of the disease.

Irrespective of the above factors, some individuals appear to be more infectious, and some more vulnerable to infection, than others. This may be because HIV frequently mutates into slightly different forms, some of which appear to be more harmful and to replicate more quickly than others.

Poverty both creates the conditions which facilitate the spread of HIV/AIDS and prevents an effective response

The Price of Poverty

With certain exceptions, the overriding reason for the rapid spread of HIV has been the high correlation that exists between poverty and vulnerability to the virus, a correlation that has led to high rates of infection in the most economically deprived populations of cities as far apart as Bombay, Edinburgh, New York and Rio de Janeiro.

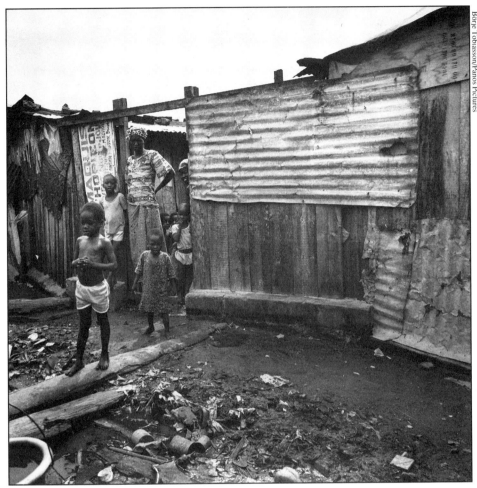

Börje Tobiasson/Panos Pictures

Abidjan, Côte d'Ivoire. The poor are the hardest hit: low levels of literacy, health and income make it harder for communities to reduce the spread of HIV/AIDS.

Poor communities have less access to health care. STDs are widespread in many developing countries because individuals cannot afford treatment, and health authorities cannot afford to provide the comprehensive network of clinics and medical staff that would ensure disease prevention and care.

Poor people tend to receive less education and are therefore more likely to be illiterate, which limits their access to information about HIV/AIDS. Illiteracy may be compounded by lack of access to radio or television. Those with little or no education tend to start their sexual life without any knowledge of the means of preventing HIV/AIDS or other STDs, or pregnancy [25]. Even where awareness of HIV/AIDS exists, people may not be able to afford condoms or there may not be the infrastructure to distribute them effectively, free or for sale.

Poverty both creates the conditions which facilitate the spread

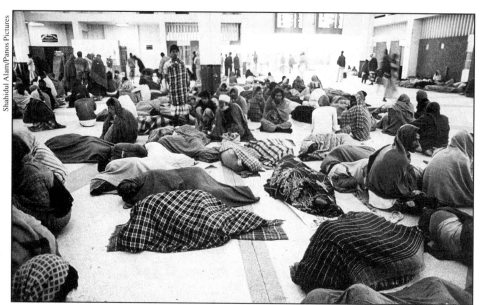

Rural migrants in search of work sleep in a railway station, Dhaka, Bangladesh. Migration breaks up families and has contributed to a rise in the number of all STDs, including HIV.

of HIV/AIDS and prevents an effective response to the epidemic. The less money available to support measures to limit the spread of HIV, the greater the likely impact of the epidemic. Access to health and education facilities has been further limited in many developing countries in the past decade by the demands of structural adjustment: policies attached to loans and imposed by the International Monetary Fund to bring about reforms in the economies of recipient countries. These reforms usually include the lessening of state controls on the economy. To qualify for these loans, governments often had to cut back on social services; as a result, spending on health and welfare fell dramatically during the 1980s. Researchers in Nigeria and Zimbabwe argue that: "Economic recession and SAPs [structural adjustment policies] further aggravate the transmission, spread and control of HIV infection in Africa in two major ways: directly by increasing the population at risk through increased urban migration, poverty, women's powerlessness and prostitution, and indirectly through a decrease in health care provision [26]."

Poverty is also forcing more and more people to leave their families and migrate in search of work. In the rural areas of developing countries, permanent and seasonal migration to urban and industrial centres or to other countries is increasing. This disruption to social and family patterns has implications for the spread of HIV.

Poverty also affects attitudes to risk-taking. To people

Migration and population movement

Because HIV is passed from person to person, it is closely associated with the movement of people from place to place [49]. Throughout the developing world, limited opportunities for employment, particularly in rural areas, have contributed to permanent and seasonal urban migration, both within countries and across frontiers. In many parts of Africa the pattern of industrial development has been based largely on male migrant labour. In several Asian countries, many young people leave rural areas to find work in urban areas or abroad, often the oil-rich states of the Gulf. In 1991, 70,000 Thai labourers travelled abroad to find employment, sending home nearly $1 billion in wages to their families [48]. Each year an estimated 5-6 million people migrate, legally or illegally, from Latin America and the Caribbean to the United States in search of employment. Migration in some areas is seen almost as a right of passage, with young men routinely spending a few years in distant cities before returning to settle in their rural home.

Long separations cause a breakdown in family patterns, and contributed to a rise in prostitution and the incidence of sexually transmitted diseases long before HIV appeared. Men who contract an STD put their partners at risk on return visits to their homes. More recently, male migration has been matched by that of single women who, with no means of support in their villages, move to the cities. Most migrants aim for regular employment; if unsuccessful, women may end up working as prostitutes. For others, such as the thousands of young women migrating from the hills of Nepal to the cities of India, prostitution is recognised as the only option. Various studies have confirmed the link between migration and the spread of HIV infection [50]. Migrants who contract HIV abroad may return home voluntarily or as the result of deportation. The home community must then compensate for the lost income and find the resources to care for the sick person. Population mobility also stems from other factors: trade and business travel (long-distance lorry-drivers have been identified as a high risk group, for example), tourism, and war and destabilisation. During periods of civil insecurity, social norms are disrupted, families are broken up, soldiers are constantly on the move, incidents of rape increase and in general there tend to be increases in the spread of all STDs.

struggling to meet their immediate needs for food and shelter, avoiding a disease which might not materialise for years can be low on their list of priorities. As Mazuwa Banda of the Churches Medical Association of Zambia points out: "There is the feeling that life is already hard. There are other priorities like getting the next meal which press on people much more than AIDS. They first want to secure food and housing before they can think of AIDS. And the long incubation period makes them think of it as a problem of tomorrow, not today [27]."

In addition, alcohol, drugs and sex are sometimes the only means of escape from a harsh existence. Once AIDS has entered this vicious circle, it intensifies dramatically. A study carried out in the Rakai district of Uganda, which has been devastated by the combination of HIV/AIDS following on from the civil war, found that some men resorted to heavy drinking as a way of forgetting

The poorer a woman, the less chance she has to protect herself

their poverty and depression. As Ugandan journalist David Musoke explains, some of these then sleep with women whose husbands have died of AIDS and who have resorted to brewing as one of the few economic options available. Those men are likely to infect their wives, which leads to more of the "sickness and death which is the main cause of their depression....As a result, men in Rakai district are trapped in a vicious circle of poverty, booze and AIDS". (See Chapter 4, p50.)

The Gender Gap

Poverty breeds powerlessness—the inability to control one's own life. And the poorest of the world's poor tend to be women. They are also the most disadvantaged by social and cultural notions of what is acceptable behaviour, sexual and otherwise. The result is that across the world, women's inferior economic and social status directly increases their vulnerability to HIV, and limits their ability to control their sex lives and protect themselves.

In most countries, formal and informal discrimination prevent all but a minority of women from achieving higher education or well-paid jobs. Low levels of female literacy are common. In some countries women are hardly represented in the formal workforce: for example, only 6.5% of Bangladesh's formal workforce is female [28]. The result is that the majority of women, especially those of child-bearing age, are economically dependent on men.

This dependence frequently reduces women's ability to determine the terms on which they have sex, including whether a condom is used and whether their regular partner is sexually faithful. In the words of Elizabeth Ngugi, lecturer at the University of Nairobi's Department of Community Health, women's poor bargaining position "leaves [them] in a state of conditioned helplessness to say no to unprotected sex [29]". And while infidelity is by no means exclusive to men, in most societies it is far more acceptable for a man to have more than one regular partner. In one Rwandan study, most women who were infected were monogamous and had contracted HIV from their non-monogamous partners [30]. This picture is repeated elsewhere. In Colombia, for example, and in other Latin American countries, the group of women most at risk are the monogamous wives of men with several sexual partners.

Economic dependence may also determine with whom a woman has sex. In extreme economic hardship a woman may offer sexual intercourse in return for support for herself and her

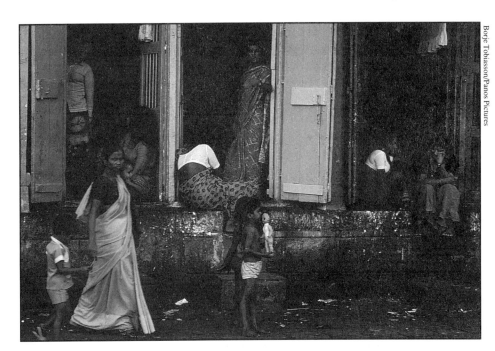

Borje Tobiasson/Panos Pictures

The "red light" district, Bombay. It is not prostitution per se which spreads HIV/AIDS but a prostitute's lack of power to dictate the terms of her trade. Poorer prostitutes show higher levels of infection than their richer counterparts.

children; the term prostitution is often misapplied in such circumstances, since neither partner may regard the relationship in this light. More clearly defined prostitution—in which sex is sold to clients for money—is a huge industry employing millions of women worldwide. For many, it is the only means of economic survival.

The number of sexual partners a woman has, therefore, is frequently determined by her low economic status, while for a man to have more than one regular or casual partner is not only usually by choice rather than circumstance, it can be a kind of status symbol. It is also facilitated by a man's greater ability to control his own life, financially and socially.

The poorer a woman, the less chance she has to protect herself. This is borne out by high infection rates among poorer women with many sexual partners. One survey in Nairobi showed women prostitutes of lower socio-economic status were more than twice as likely to be infected than prostitutes of higher socio-economic status [31]. Infection rates among women prostitutes in the urban slums of India are rising rapidly. Tests carried out on nearly 2,000 women working in Bombay's "red light" areas between September 1986 and January 1990 revealed a rapid increase in HIV infections—from very few women initially, to almost one-quarter in the six-month period up to January 1990 [32].

The poor are the most vulnerable, but by no means the only targets of the disease

In sub-Saharan Africa, further evidence of the inequality between the sexes is revealed by the average age at which men and women contract HIV, as older men put pressure on younger women to have intercourse. Infection amongst women rises rapidly as teenagers begin sexual activity, reaching a peak in the 20-30 age group. In men, HIV prevalence is highest in the 25-35 age group   [33]. There have been increasing reports of men seeking very young partners whom they assume to be free of infection, while "some male secondary school teachers stated that sex is one of the fringe benefits of a poorly paid profession [34]". Finally, women who wish to conceive cannot practise safe sex.

Thus the economic and social inequalities associated with gender, together with the physical factors described earlier, mean that women are more vulnerable to all STDs, including HIV. According to WHO, over 15,000 women become infected with HIV every week, and in more and more countries the male to female infection rate is drawing closer to one to one [35].

A dynamic situation

In the early 1990s, the global picture presented by HIV/AIDS is that of a series of concurrent sub-epidemics striking different population groups with different intensities. It is a dynamic situation where the poor and the marginalised are the most vulnerable, but by no means the only, targets of the disease. Broadly speaking, the deeper a woman's poverty, the greater her vulnerability, while in the early stages of the epidemic, a man's frequently increases with his relative wealth. This early disproportionate impact on the more educated, skilled male worker has particularly significant economic implications. Yet whether infection is concentrated in the wealthier and better educated citizens or in those who are poor and less educated, HIV/AIDS threatens the overall development prospects of whole nations by primarily attacking men and women aged between 20 and 45—the backbone of the labour force.

CHAPTER 2

The demographic impact

The lengthy incubation period of HIV/AIDS means that even if all HIV transmission were to halt immediately, the number of AIDS cases would continue to grow during the next decade at an average rate of 10% a year. But because transmission will continue, 40 million people—a number that could rise to over 100 million—could have contracted the virus by the end of the century. Even the most conservative estimates predict that the number of people who will have developed or died from AIDS may reach 10 million, almost 90% of whom will be in the developing world, while as many as 10 million children will have been orphaned by the disease [1].

HIV is also causing increased illness and death among individuals who have not contracted the virus. Recent rises in the incidence of tuberculosis in sub-Saharan Africa and the United States are directly attributable to the spread of HIV infection (see Chapter 3). And studies show that uninfected children of HIV-positive mothers have higher mortality rates than the children of HIV-negative mothers.

This chapter examines the demographic background to the epidemic and the possible impact of HIV/AIDS. Exactly how many people will contract HIV and what impact their numbers will have on individual countries or communities depends on a number of factors, including how fast the epidemic spreads, which age groups and social classes are most affected and how quickly behaviour change is achieved. Mathematical models created to predict possible future paths of the epidemic come to different conclusions, according to different assumptions as to seroprevalence, rates of partner change and many other factors associated with the epidemic.

Population profiles
Variations in birth rates and life expectancies mean that population profiles—the proportion of different age groups that make up a nation's population—differ across the world. The industrialised world is characterised by low birth rates and long

Table 1: World population

	Population (billions)	Average growth rate (%)	Birth rate (per 1,000)	Life expectancy (years)	Infant mortality* (per 1,000)	Fertility (per 1,000)
World	5.3	1.7	26	66	63	3.3
More developed countries	1.2	0.5	14	75	12	1.9
Less developed countries	4.1	2.1	30	63	70	3.7
Africa	0.6	3.0	43	54	94	6.0
Latin America & the Caribbean	0.4	1.9	27	68	48	3.2
Asia	3.1	1.8	27	65	64	3.3

* under 12 months

Source: *State of World Population 1992*, UNFPA

life expectancies, which result in populations which are fairly evenly spread across the age spectrum; in many developing countries higher birth rates and lower life expectancies mean that children and young adults form a higher proportion of the population.

Fertility—the number of children a woman gives birth to—averages 3.7 in the developing world, in comparison to 1.9 in industrialised countries. Poverty is a key factor in fertility. Throughout the world poorer women tend to have more children; high fertility rates lead to higher rates of maternal and infant deaths. Each year half a million women die during pregnancy and childbirth, 99% of them in developing countries. Too frequent childbirth may lead to underweight newborns, while babies who are weaned too quickly are at risk of malnutrition if there are no alternatives to breast milk [2].

For these and other reasons child and adult mortality rates are much higher in the developing world. Child mortality (deaths in children under five) averages 112 per 1,000 live births, compared with 18 per 1,000 in the industrialised world [3]. In the developing world, about one in four people who live to the age of 15 will die before the age of 60, whereas in Japan (the country with the longest life expectancy) the rate is approximately one in nine for men and one in 16 for women [4].

Because most nations in the developing world have smaller proportions of their population in the 15-60 age group, dependency ratios—the number of children and elderly people dependent on working adults—are high. As Table 2 indicates, in Latin America and the Caribbean there are approximately 800

Table 2: Dependency ratios (per 1,000 working adults)

		Latin America/ Caribbean	Sub-Saharan Africa	Middle East/ North Africa	Asia/ Pacific	Industrialised countries
1985	Age group					
	0-14	37.6	46.0	42.7	35.0	22.1
	15-59	55.7	49.4	52.1	58.0	61.9
	60+	6.9	4.6	5.2	7.0	16.0
	Dependency ratio	**799**	**1,024**	**919**	**724**	**616**
2000*	Age group					
	0-14	31.9	45.1	41.3	30.6	19.9
	15-59	60.5	50.4	53.4	61.1	61.7
	60+	7.6	4.5	5.3	8.4	18.4
	Dependency ratio	**653**	**984**	**873**	**638**	**621**

*The figures for 2000 do not take into account the possible impact of HIV/AIDS.

Source: *The Health of Adults in the Developing World*, World Bank, May 1991. Dependency figures calculated by Panos

children and elderly people for every 1,000 working adults. In sub-Saharan Africa this rises to over 1,000 dependants, whereas in industrialised countries there are about 600. This means that when a working adult dies in sub-Saharan Africa, the number of dependants the community must support is considerably higher than elsewhere. However, dependency ratios reveal only part of the picture of a country's potential or actual workforce: they do not take account of, for example, unemployment, the incidence of child labour, the proportion of the population ill and unable to work, nor the proportion of older—and therefore more experienced and skilled—working adults.

Modelling the Epidemic

No-one can predict with certainty the full impact of the HIV/AIDS epidemic on fertility and mortality in any country—and therefore on that country's population profile. As described in Chapter 1, the sub-epidemics are the result of a number of social and physical factors. Some of these factors are known to vary considerably, while others are only now becoming the subject of detailed research. But even if present trends could be tracked with accuracy, the dynamic nature of the epidemic means that future patterns of spread may be very different. Increased drug injection using shared needles, for example, may result in faster transmission, while growing awareness of the disease may result in a significant reduction in the rate of spread.

No-one can predict with certainty the full impact of the epidemic

Most diseases strike the weakest first: the very young and the old. HIV/AIDS primarily targets adults, leaving children and the elderly without those on whom they traditionally depend.

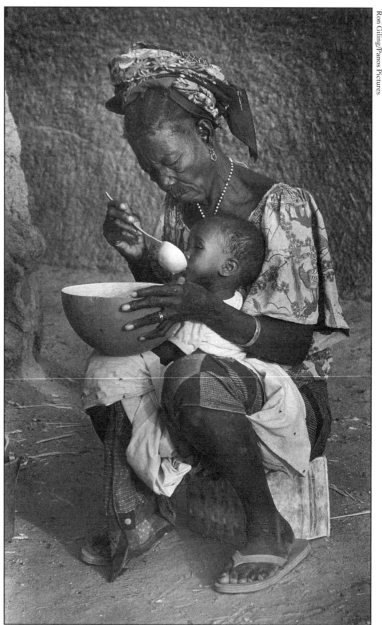

Ron Giling/Panos Pictures

A number of mathematical models have been developed which predict the likely course of the epidemic in specific countries or regions or in hypothetical populations. Most scenarios emphasise heterosexual transmission of HIV, which reflects the fact that most of the data available is on the epidemic in sub-Saharan Africa. By entering different values for such factors as current seroprevalence, efficiency of transmission and partner change, different scenarios—pictures of the future course of the epidemic—emerge. For example, the extent to which life expectancies will drop, or whether or not population size will fall, differs from scenario to scenario.

Life expectancy in sub-Saharan Africa could fall to 47 years by the end of the century

These models and the different scenarios they produce serve two purposes. One is to increase understanding of the process by which the epidemic spreads, by analysing the implications if certain things happen—for example, looking at which factors seem to lead to greater increases in infection—or if certain courses of action are taken. The second is to serve as an instrument for policymakers by depicting possible impacts of HIV/AIDS. But any picture offered by a model must be treated with care, because it is not a prediction of what the future must be but only one possible scenario out of many [5].

One picture of the epidemic that has emerged from several models is that of "waves" representing the spread of infection from a small high risk group, who do not use condoms and who frequently change sexual partners, to others in the community. The first wave produces a rapidly developing but relatively small epidemic of very high levels of infection in the high risk group; the second wave is a more slowly developing but much larger epidemic in the majority of the population. The interval between these two waves may be several decades [6]. This would suggest that even in the worst affected countries, the HIV/AIDS epidemic is still in its early stages.

Adult mortality

Within 10 years of its discovery in 1981, HIV/AIDS has had a significant impact on mortality rates in a number of countries, becoming one of the leading causes of death in the 20-40 age group in major cities in the Americas, Western Europe and sub-Saharan Africa [7]. Adult death rates in East and Central Africa are roughly 1.3%; one scenario suggests that, 25 years after the start of the epidemic, AIDS deaths may cause this to rise by a further 1.3% [8].

WHO, referring to a model developed at the World Bank, says life expectancy in sub-Saharan Africa could fall to 47 years by the end of the century, in place of the 62 years expected in the absence of HIV/AIDS [9]. This assumes infection rates of 40% [10]. A model devised by Roy Anderson and associates at Imperial College, London (the "Anderson model") concludes that a 20-year-old man in sub-Saharan Africa has an 87% expectancy of reaching 40 in the absence of HIV, a rate which falls to under 75% when average HIV infection rates in the general population

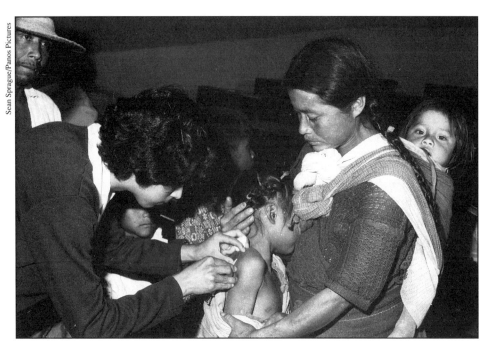

Sean Sprague/Panos Pictures

Chiapas, Mexico. Immunisation and improved living standards have reduced levels of child mortality in many developing countries. These gains may be reversed by HIV/AIDS.

reach 1%. When infection rates reach 5%, as has already happened in some countries, his chances of reaching 40 are no greater than 50% [11].

Child mortality

The impact of HIV/AIDS on child mortality is likely to reverse the gains made since the early 1960s in many developing countries by immunisation programmes and improving living standards. UNICEF, the United Nations Children's Fund, predicts that the under-five mortality rate in Central and East Africa, instead of dropping to around 132 deaths per 1,000 live births as earlier projected, is likely to rise to between 159 and 189 per 1,000 [12], with up to 500,000 deaths occurring annually by the end of the century [13]. WHO predicts that wherever female infection rates are high, child mortality could be as much as 30% greater than would otherwise have been expected [14]. The organisation also predicts that before the mid-1990s AIDS will cause more deaths in children in sub-Saharan Africa than either malaria or measles [15].

In addition to children dying of AIDS, there is evidence of higher mortality in the HIV-negative children of HIV-positive mothers. These children are often already underweight and less healthy than babies born to HIV-negative mothers [16]. Because of her illness, a mother with HIV/AIDS appears to place her child at increased risk of being malnourished, and of contracting endemic infections such as tuberculosis; ultimately, such a child is more likely to be orphaned, further reducing his/her access to care.

Fertility

Many of the social and physical factors associated with gender combine to concentrate HIV infection in young women of child-bearing age. Whether this will lead to a net rise or fall in births—and what proportion of newborns will be HIV-negative —is as yet unclear. The long incubation period of the disease means that the opportunities for many HIV-positive women to have children will not be reduced. On the other hand, the epidemic has the potential to reduce fertility if a smaller proportion of the population survives to child-bearing age. Furthermore, increased condom use will have the side effect of preventing some unintended pregnancies [17].

Perceptions of HIV and the risk of infection may, therefore, have as strong an influence on fertility as seroprevalence rates. According to Maxine Ankrah, of Makerere University, Uganda: "Women of childbearing age are caught in a particular dilemma...heightened anxiety, guilt, fear and depression [follow] an HIV/AIDS diagnosis....Because most African cultures expect all women to bear children, failure to do so is tantamount to inviting social ridicule and humiliation, if not divorce or displacement in the marital union."

Ankrah also says that there is anecdotal evidence that "women may be having more pregnancies to offset the perceived threat of infant mortality—and to ensure the survival of at least some offspring [18]."

An Uncertain Picture

It is uncertain how much the changes in mortality rates and possible changes in fertility rates induced by HIV/AIDS will affect population size and population profiles. Most scenarios depict no more than a slowing in the population growth rate as the epidemic spreads, although one produced by the Anderson model suggests a decline in population after 30 years if seroprevalence in the sexually active population, both urban and rural, reaches 35%-40% [19]. However, it is arguable that behaviour change is likely to occur long before such levels of seroprevalence are reached.

Another area of uncertainty is whether rural rates of infection will remain low (mostly under 5%) or reach the urban levels of 25%-33% of the worst-affected countries. In rural Zaire, for example, infection rates did not increase in the 10-year period from the mid-1970s to the mid-1980s [20], and in other parts of the continent rural rates remained static even at the end of the 1980s [21]. It has been suggested that HIV prevalence may remain low in most rural areas because sexual activity is more restricted in terms of potential partner change. In this respect, population mobility is a key factor and areas where there is a regular pattern of rural-urban migration are likely to see higher rates. Overall, it may be that levels of HIV infection in rural areas will rise only when a critical, and as yet undetermined, rate is reached in urban settings.

Most models predict little overall change in dependency ratios as a result of the epidemic. However, this picture of relative stability is likely to mask some significant shifts in the population profile. According to the Anderson model, increasing severity of the epidemic leads to increased deaths of mature adults and so to a rise in the proportion of the population aged 15 to 25, rising to 33% in the worst scenario. This compares with 19% in the absence of HIV [22]. This means that, while the overall

Regional predictions

In 1992, WHO predicted that up to 40 million people worldwide would have contracted HIV by the end of the century. For the same date, the Global AIDS Policy Coalition, an independent institute based in the United States, predicted that 110 million people would be infected. Although there may be disagreement about overall numbers, there is general agreement as to the pattern of the pandemic that will develop.

In industrialised countries, the decline in the rate of homosexual transmission is likely to continue, while transmission through injecting drug use will increase, leading to a slow increase in heterosexual transmission.

In sub-Saharan Africa, the pattern of heterosexual transmission will continue, leading to high numbers of children infected.

In Latin America and the Caribbean, the proportion of cases resulting from heterosexual transmission will continue to grow. Changes in drug-taking behaviour may lead to faster spread of the epidemic if shared needle use becomes widespread.

In South and Southeast Asia the epidemic "may be growing at a pace reminiscent of sub-Saharan Africa in the early 1980s but may have an even greater potential for spread, given the adult population of nearly 500 million as compared with 225 million in sub-Saharan Africa [33]." Heterosexual spread will be the main mode of transmission.

In Central and Eastern Europe, and the republics of the former USSR, there is considerable potential for rapid spread of HIV. The political upheavals of recent years have affected health infrastructures, while the abolition of travel restrictions and greater political freedom may have social consequences that include greater opportunity for sexual contact with foreigners and access to injectable drugs.

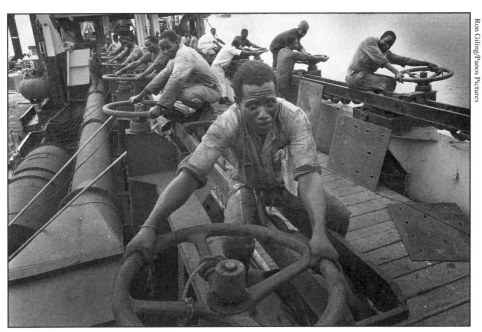

Ron Giling/Panos Pictures

*Maputo,
Mozambique.
HIV/AIDS has a
particularly deadly
characteristic: it
strikes the
backbone of a
country's labour
force, men and
women aged
between 20 and 45.*

dependency ratio would not change, the burden would increasingly fall on the younger, inexperienced adults.

The other problem with this overall picture of stable dependency ratios is that, like all averages, it obscures what is happening at the individual level. The mathematical predictions appear to conflict with actual reports of thousands of children left orphaned in the worst affected countries of sub-Saharan Africa. A possible, unconfirmed explanation of this apparent contradiction is that in areas in which many children have lost one or both parents, many adults have lost children to the disease. If the number of orphans approximated the number of additional child deaths, there would be no change to dependency ratios, as the models predict, although there would be many children left orphaned and many bereaved parents [23].

The future trend is unclear. Scenarios produced by the Anderson model predict that the long-term impact of the epidemic will be to reduce the proportion of children in the population [24]; this suggests that the orphan burden will be reduced as the birth rate falls, as children with HIV die and as children without HIV outgrow their orphan status. A model devised by the US Interagency Working Group and coordinated by the US Bureau of the Census (the "IWG model") suggests the opposite: as adult mortality continues to rise so will the number of orphans [25].

The Impact of Interventions

Most experts believe that there will be some change in behaviour as a result of HIV/AIDS—such as fewer sexual partners and increased condom use—but none can predict with certainty the extent of such change. All agree, however, that the effectiveness of reducing heterosexual spread of the virus depends to a large extent on which point in the history of the epidemic measures to achieve behaviour change are introduced. As examined in Chapter 8, the higher the infection rate when behaviour change starts, the more deep-rooted the epidemic and its economic and social effects and the more difficult it is for such change to have an impact.

Most mathematical models describe a number of scenarios which take behaviour change into account. The IWG model predicts that a 5% reduction in the number of casual sexual contacts in urban areas would result in average urban infection reaching 12% rather than 17% by 2015, while a 20% or greater reduction would result in a decline in overall infection rates [26]. A study based on the IWG model and commissioned for the Thai government (the "Thai study") predicts that reducing sexual contacts with different partners by 50%, doubling condom use from 25% to 50% and rapidly and effectively treating sexually transmitted diseases would cause overall rates of HIV infection to remain static, with the result that 3.5 million fewer people would be infected by the year 2000 [27].

Reducing transmission in the section of the population at highest risk is likely to have a far greater effect than reducing transmission among people who change sexual partners infrequently. A World Bank paper compared the impact of preventing cases of HIV and other STDs of equivalent numbers in these two groups. Preventing 100 cases of HIV among the highly active population resulted in the prevention of 10-20 new cases of HIV a month over 10 years; preventing 100 cases in the less sexually active population resulted in the prevention of under five new cases a month. The paper concluded that, depending on the incidence of genital ulcers, preventing transmission of HIV infection in the highly sexually active population has up to 10 times more impact than in the less active population. Similar figures hold true for prevention of other sexually transmitted diseases [28].

Treatment

There is little evidence to suggest that the rise in HIV/AIDS-related deaths in the developing world will be mitigated in the near to medium future by improved treatment for the disease. Health care professionals are gaining experience in treating opportunistic infections, which allows the average period from diagnosis of AIDS to death to lengthen, although even in the industrialised world such improvement is in terms of months rather than years. Anti-viral drugs can postpone development of AIDS in people who are HIV-positive and have not yet developed symptoms, but the cost of such treatment places it beyond reach of almost all those infected in the developing world.

There is still great potential to influence the future course of the epidemic

It has been suggested that if treatment to prolong life were widely available in the developing world, this might lead to further spread of the epidemic as there would be a longer period for those who were HIV-positive to pass on the infection to others [29]. This assumes, however, that those who received treatment would continue to infect others. Such a scenario is unlikely, given that most people do not wish to infect others, and in communities where such treatment were available, adequate counselling and resources for prevention and education would also probably be available and so would significantly reduce HIV transmission.

Optimism and pessimism
The range of predictions on a global scale has been matched on a country level by sometimes apocalyptic visions of HIV/AIDS-induced population decline. The more extreme predictions are unlikely to come to pass, since they are based on the premise that no behaviour change has taken or will take place. Nonetheless, the potential for further widespread dissemination of HIV can be seen in the more than 200 million new cases of sexually transmitted diseases that appear in the world each year. Indeed, the incidence of existing STDs offers a rough indication of a country's level of vulnerability—as India, for example, has discovered to its cost. Despite high rates of STDs in the 1980s, many Indians predicted that HIV/AIDS would remain a "foreign disease". The reality now is that it has taken root in the country's cities and has been detected in almost every state. In the 1990s, China, with a fifth of the world's population, is in a similar position: HIV infection rates are low but, despite official disapproval of pre-marital and non-monogamous sexual activity, STD rates have been rising steeply in recent years. Bangladesh, similarly, has low rates of HIV infection, but one of the highest rates of genital ulcers in women worldwide, which significantly increases their vulnerability to the epidemic [30].

Jonathan Mann, ex-director of WHO's Global Programme on AIDS and currently director of the Harvard International AIDS

WHO
continues to
revise its
predictions
upwards

Center, points out that: "The most important feature of the HIV pandemic is that it is still at a relatively early stage of its development. This has three consequences: first, the pandemic remains volatile and dynamic; second, its major impact has yet to be felt; and third, there is still great potential to influence its future course [31]."

Mann's conclusion, shared by most researchers, that the different HIV epidemics across the world are only in their early stages, gives grounds for both pessimism and optimism. Pessimism, because the potential for further spread of the virus, with concomitant illness, poverty and death, remains high. Optimism, because there remains scope for action to limit the spread.

But if there is optimism and pessimism, they are sharply divided between the industrialised and developing worlds. In countries such as Australia and the United Kingdom, changes in behaviour by homosexual men have meant that levels of infection and numbers of cases of AIDS in the early 1990s have not reached the high levels predicted in the mid-1980s. In most parts of the world, however, and particularly in Asia, where action taken in the mid-1980s might have reduced some of the present impact of the disease, the numbers of those infected and affected continues to rise. WHO continues to revise its predictions—considered conservative by some—upwards not downwards (in 1988 the organisation predicted 18 million infections by the end of the century [32]; four years later that figure had risen to 30-40 million), and repeats that by the year 2000, 90% of all those who have contracted HIV will be in the developing world. The possible social and economic consequences of such a scenario are described in the following chapters.

CHAPTER 3

Health costs

In 1990, the cost of treatment for the global total of people with AIDS—some 200,000-330,000 patients—was estimated at between $2.6 billion and $3.5 billion. Although not more than 40% of all AIDS cases that year were in the industrialised world, they accounted for 84% of all expenditure. No more than 2% of spending was in Africa, which had 50% of all people with AIDS. In every country surveyed, hospital care was the major cost [1].

These figures illustrate how the treatment received by patients with AIDS reflects above all the resources available—and the resources available for health care vary dramatically between North and South. Even in the North, the system is under pressure, particularly in the United States, where lack of a national health system means many patients with HIV, but without insurance or entitlement to health care benefits, receive inadequate treatment. In many developing countries, the demands of structural adjustment policies have already forced governments to reduce public spending on health. Countries such as Thailand and India with high rates of HIV infection but as yet few cases of AIDS face potentially very high costs in the next five to ten years. In those developing countries where the HIV/AIDS epidemic has been extant for 10 or more years, the ability of individuals and already overstretched health systems to cope with the disease is under severe strain. In parts of sub-Saharan Africa one in four hospital beds is occupied by a patient being treated for symptoms associated with HIV, while the costs of palliative treatment alone are far beyond the $5 or less per person per year that countries in the region have available for medical care.

The direct costs of HIV/AIDS

Any endemic or epidemic disease places a burden on a country's health budget. The economic costs of a disease are generally estimated as the **direct costs** of medical care and the **indirect costs** of labour—and therefore potential income—lost because of illness and death of patients and the task of caring for patients. Indirect costs are explored in Chapters 5 and 6.

*Two per cent
of spending
on AIDS
treatment was
in Africa,
which had
50% of all
people with
AIDS*

Direct costs include all the hospital costs of doctors, nurses, drugs, equipment, administration and so on, as well as the costs of out-of-hospital care, such as hospices, health visitors and counselling. HIV/AIDS, a disease characterised by intermittent bouts of illness, places particular demands on hospitals, medical staff and health budgets.

An Unequal Picture

In the late 1980s, a rough calculation shows that, on average, $1,250 was spent per person per year on health care in the industrialised world, compared with $35 in Latin America and the Caribbean, and under $5 in both South Asia and sub-Saharan Africa [2]. Although some costs, such as salaries and administration, are lower in the developing world, these figures amply demonstrate the imbalance in the health care available in different regions of the world. Such averages mask wide variations within regions: Table 1 gives more detailed figures.

The amount of money spent on medical drugs—which reflects availability of the drugs and of the money to buy them—is a key component of these figures. While the cost of drugs varies little across the world, annual per capita drug consumption in industrialised countries in 1985 was estimated at $62, whereas in the developing world it was $5.40 [3]. Many countries in

Table 1: Health expenditure per capita (US$)

Country	1980-82	1983-85	1986-87
AFRICA			
Botswana	19	17	32
Zambia	23	8	5
Malawi	3	4	3
Kenya	9	6	6
Uganda	1	1	1
LATIN AMERICA			
Mexico	12	8	7
Peru	13	11	10
Venezuela	110	73	79
Belize	3	2	6
Brazil	152	214	207
ASIA			
Singapore	85	129	96
Thailand	8	10	10
Nepal	1	2	.1
India	1	1	1
Bangladesh	1	1	—

Source:*1991 World Health Statistics Annual*, WHO

Table 2 : Ratio of population to doctors and nurses in developing world (1984 figures)

Country	Number of people per doctor	per nurse
AFRICA		
Botswana	6,900	700
Nigeria	7,990	1,020
Zambia	7,150	740
Sudan	10,100	1,250
Kenya	9,970	950
Rwanda	34,680	3,650
LATIN AMERICA		
& the CARIBBEAN		
Honduras	1,510	670
Haiti	7,180	2,290
Venezuela	700	—
Brazil	1,080	1,210
Jamaica	2,040	490
Guatemala	2,180	850
ASIA		
Singapore	1,310	—
Thailand	6,290	710
Nepal	32,710	4,680
China	1,000	1,710
India	2,520	1,700
Bangladesh	6,730	8,980

Source: Based on figures in *Human Development Report 1992*, UNDP

sub-Saharan Africa spend much less than this figure; only one-third of the population in the region has access to such basic drugs as chloroquine or penicillin [4]. The lack of financial resources is exacerbated by lack of human resources. In most countries of the industrialised world there is one doctor for every 500 people—the corresponding figure for Mexico is 1,240; for Sri Lanka, 5,520; for Uganda, 21,900; and for Rwanda, 34,680 [5]. Whereas almost everyone in industrialised countries has access to health services, this figure drops to 93% in Sri Lanka, 78% in Mexico, 60% in Uganda and 28% in Rwanda [6].

Finance affects the quality of care available. The facilities of a typical Paris or Sydney hospital, which include consultants of every speciality, the most modern technology and a wide range of drugs, are a far cry from the Central African hospital where power cuts are frequent, drug supplies are meagre and food has to be provided by patients' relatives. A similar situation prevails in other developing countries such as Nepal, where "all kinds of treatment are available only in theory" and "public hospitals

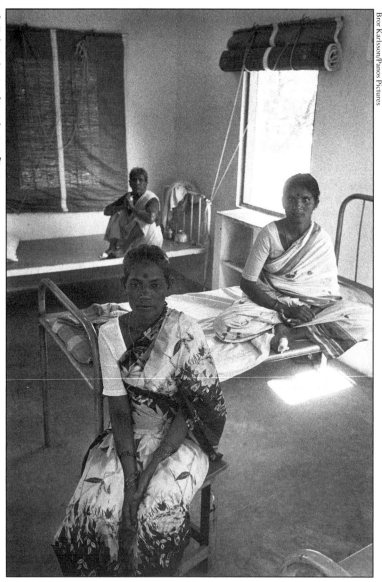

The care given to people with HIV/AIDS reflects the resources available. This hospital in Sri Lanka, a country with relatively well developed health system, has far fewer resources than a hospital in an industrialised country.

Bror Karlsson/Panos Pictures

provide very cheap and poor food, inadequate for patients' needs"
and only a few basic medicines such as aspirin are available free
[7]. Greater resources mean better hospital care (see Box
opposite), but few public hospitals in the developing world can
provide the level of care available in the North.

Treatment costs

Whatever the illness, the extent and cost of treatment a patient
receives usually depends on the national resources available,
except where individuals can afford private treatment. HIV/AIDS
is no exception. In many developing countries, treatment for

Hospital care in Chile

The Chilean health system, despite its considerable deficiencies, can provide a range of treatments for people with HIV/AIDS—if health professionals can overcome their fears and prejudices towards the patient. Chile has 14,800 doctors, 61% of whom reside and work in the capital city; the three major metropolitan areas account for 80% of all the doctors. There are about 8,000 nurses and 13,000 public and private hospital beds.

State hospitals are available to those enrolled in the state medical system through their employment or because of poverty. Those in the latter category do not pay, while others pay a percentage of costs and fees. Hospitals provide meals and their sanitary and hygienic standards are among the highest in South America.

Treatment for HIV/AIDS has improved since the first cases appeared in 1984, stimulating sensational headlines and morbid curiosity among hospital staff, but little in the way of medical care. The Arriaran Centre, informally connected to a Santiago hospital, was established in 1990 with private funds and now treats 300 patients with HIV/AIDS.

Arriaran social worker Margarita Valdes, one of the founders of the centre, says clients and their immediate family members receive full medical and dental care, psychological and nutritional counselling and hospitalisation, including free medicines. They can even get scanners and obstetric care if necessary. But patients do not have access to the more expensive AIDS-related medicines such as zidovudine.

Valdes says the centre's resources are quickly eaten up by the cost of medicines that are available and the costs of supplying these are rising steadily as new patients pour in. By the end of 1992 the intake rate is expected to rise to 10 clients a week. "We are reaching our capacity limit," says the social worker, noting that government support to the Arriaran project has been virtually nil.

Almost all public health professionals recognise that the public sector is severely underfunded. Arrarian has therefore to resist a tendency on the part of other hospitals to duck the problem by sending patients with HIV/AIDS to the centre. "We don't turn anyone away, but we encourage other hospitals to assume their responsibilities," says Valdes.

Tim Frasca, *Santiago*

people with HIV is generally restricted to those who are seriously ill, and may extend no further than palliative care. Only rarely are anti-viral drugs available. By contrast, in the industrialised world a sophisticated combination of drugs can help patients recover from many serious opportunistic infections, while anti-virals are often available for those with HIV but otherwise healthy, as an experimental means of postponing AIDS.

It is possible to look at the disparity between treatment costs in different countries, but because the basis on which figures are calculated varies, comparisons must be seen as general rather than exact [8]. For example, "lifetime costs" generally means two years in industrialised countries and one year in most developing countries, since patients in the North tend to live longer after diagnosis of AIDS.

The average lifetime cost of treating a person who has developed AIDS in the United States in 1992 was calculated as $102,000. This compares with $52,000 for breast cancer but $175,000 for kidney disease. The $102,000 is considerably higher than earlier estimates ($85,000 in 1991 and $57,000 in 1988), because many more people are receiving treatment, particularly anti-viral drugs, in the early stages of HIV disease [9].

Spending on AIDS is much lower in developing countries. Figures reported in 1988 cited lifetime direct medical costs as $132-$1,585 in Zaire and $104-$631 in Tanzania [10]. These figures represent from 0.2% to 3% of US costs in the same year. Figures given in 1989 for lifetime costs per patient ranged from $160 in Malawi, $230-$250 in Uganda and Burundi, and over $1,800 for Brazil [11]. Lifetime costs for Thailand were estimated in 1991 as $923-$1,522 [12]. Figures for the Americas range from $1,560 in Chile (presumed annual cost, exclusive of anti-viral drugs) [13], to $4,400 in Mexico (presumed lifetime costs) and $4,550 in Barbados (lifetime medical costs) [14]. A more recent (1992) study of Brazilian costs gave $8,382 as the yearly cost of a patient with AIDS [15]. For a regional summary of average annual expenditure, see Table 3.

As is the case with overall health expenditure, drugs form a major part of the HIV/AIDS figures. A patient's drug bill in the United States may be well over $1,000 a month, given that the weekly cost of some drugs reaches $200 (for example, EPO—used to treat anaemia) or even $1,000 (G-CSF—used to

Table 3: Estimated global costs of AIDS care in 1992 by region

Region	Person-years of care	Percentage of overall person-years	Cost per person-year of care (1990 $US)	Total cost of adult care (1990 million $US)	Percentage of global costs
North America	74,000	17.1	31,995	2,368	67.5
Western Europe	38,000	8.8	22,391	851	24.3
Oceania	1,600	0.4	14,015	22	0.6
Latin America	33,000	7.6	1,992	66	1.9
Africa	254,000	58.7	393	100	2.8
Caribbean	10,000	2.3	2,157	22	0.6
Eastern Europe	1,500	0.3	1,520	2	0.1
Southeast Mediterranean	1,000	0.2	2,446	2	0.1
Northeast Asia	1,800	0.4	23,160	42	1.2
Southeast Asia	18,000	4.2	1,700	31	0.9
TOTAL	432,900	100.0		3,506	100.0

Source: Taken from *AIDS in the World 1992*, Global AIDS Policy Coalition, Harvard University

Zidovudine

Despite the financial burden, there is increasing but limited use of zidovudine (AZT), ddI (Didanosine) and other anti-viral drugs in the developing world, usually on research basis. Zidovudine, which was first given to patients with AIDS in 1987, has proved effective in prolonging the lives of those who have developed AIDS. Studies suggest it is also effective in postponing the onset of symptoms in those who are HIV-positive [47]. The annual cost of an average dose of zidovudine is $1,200 (based on the dose of five capsules a day at $1.20 per capsule). The average cost of ddI is $40 a week [48].

However, to put the potential use of such drugs into perspective, the Pan American Health Organization calculated that to provide zidovudine for the 12,000 people living with AIDS in Latin America in 1990 would have cost almost $32 million a year. The combined budget for prevention and care activities by National AIDS Programmes in the region in the same year was estimated at under $13 million [49]. To provide zidovudine for the 1 million individuals estimated to have HIV in Latin America would cost almost $3 billion [50].

If the one million individuals in Uganda believed to be HIV-positive were to be given zidovudine, the total annual cost would be $1.2 billion, 100 times the country's annual health expenditure and eight times the country's annual export earnings [51]. Moreover, estimates of the costs of zidovudine generally exclude the time and equipment involved in closely monitoring individuals' health, which is a prerequisite of prescribing the drug.

treat low white blood cell count or neutropenia) [16]. This figure contrasts with the average lifetime drug costs for a person with AIDS in Zambia of $30-$40, where the highest percentage (28%) comes from drugs used for tuberculosis [17]. Drug costs for Thailand are estimated as $60-$90 per patient per year [18].

Although there are huge discrepancies in treatment costs between countries, within many developing countries some patients with HIV/AIDS do not necessarily incur higher hospital costs than other patients. One Zaire hospital study indicated that on average HIV-positive patients did not differ significantly from other patients in total spending or length of stay. This was largely because the hospital studied was inadequately equipped to diagnose and treat HIV-related diseases—so again this was a reflection of the limits to available resources.

However, the picture is complicated by two factors: that this calculation does not include the higher medical costs for people with HIV before hospitalisation, and that the high percentage of HIV-positive patients who died reduced the average costs of hospitalisation. If these factors are taken into account, overall medical costs in the Zaire study were higher—$170 for HIV-positive patients and $110 for HIV-negative patients, and length of hospital stay longer—25 days for HIV-positive patients and 18 days for HIV-negative patients [19].

The Cost of Tuberculosis

Tuberculosis (TB)—one of the commonest opportunistic infections to which HIV-positive people are prone—has a significant impact on costs. Preliminary results from ADZAM, a study of the economic aspects of adult disease in Zambia, showed that patients with HIV but without TB stayed only slightly longer (11 days) than those with neither infection (9 days). Patients with both HIV and TB stayed nearly twice as long (21 days) as those with HIV and no TB [20]. A Congo study gave average length of stay for patients with HIV and TB as 44 days in comparison with 36 for those with TB alone [21]. A similar impact has been seen in the United States: a study in New York, where HIV-related TB cases rose from 71 in 1983 to 3,496 in 1990, showed that patients with TB and HIV were hospitalised for 31 days compared with 20 days for those with HIV and other infections [22].

ADZAM calculates the average cost per hospital stay of people in Zambia with HIV but without TB as $39, similar to the average of $41 for patients with neither infection. It is the length of stay and the drugs required by TB patients which increase the medical costs. The average cost of a stay in the TB ward for patients irrespective of HIV status, including diagnostics and drugs, was $115, equivalent to $5.50 a day [23]. A similar figure—

Figure 1: How TB affects length of hospital stay: two examples

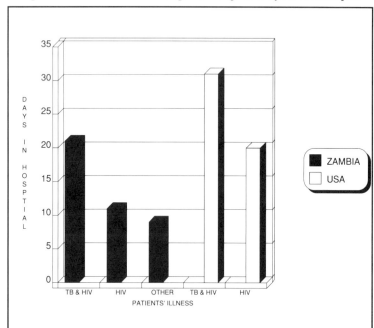

TB is the most important AIDS-associated infection in the world

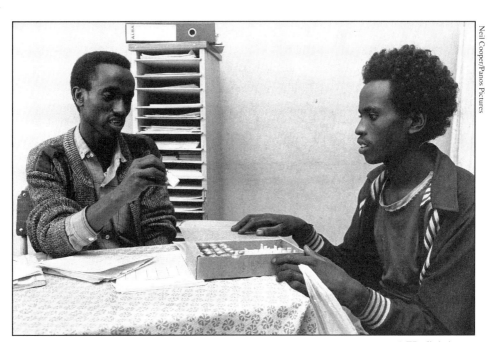

Neil Cooper/Panos Pictures

$126—has been given for Uganda [24].

The HIV/AIDS epidemic is also increasing illness in people who have not contracted the virus. As more people with HIV contract TB, the disease becomes more widespread and there is a higher incidence among people who are HIV-negative. As with HIV/AIDS, mortality from TB is highest in the 15-59 age group.

A TB clinic in Ethiopia: developing countries are facing an accelerating epidemic of TB and HIV co-infection.

Falling costs?

Tuberculosis aside, some of the medical costs of HIV/AIDS in the early 1990s may be falling. In both industrialised and developing countries, greater familiarity with the symptoms presented by the disease has allowed doctors to treat patients with greater efficiency, even where resources are severely restricted, thus allowing many to spend less time in hospital. In one Mexican hospital, for example, length of stay fell by 34% between 1990 and 1991 thanks to more efficient outpatient care [25].

On the other hand, the extended lifespan of many people with AIDS, particularly in the industrialised world, may lead to higher costs per patient. In the UK, the proportion of people living for at least two years after diagnosis of AIDS rose between 1984 and 1988 from under 20% to more than 45% [26]. Above all, while the average length of hospital stay of HIV-positive patients decreases, the rising number of those infected will draw ever more heavily on national health resources.

A dangerous liaison: HIV and TB

The developing world is confronting a massive and accelerating epidemic of TB and HIV co-infection. WHO estimates that 4.5 million people, 98% of them in the developing world, are co-infected. This is almost certainly an underestimate.

The economic and social implications of tuberculosis (TB) and HIV co-infection are grave. Paul Nunn, of the London School of Hygiene and Tropical Medicine, says the risk groups for both epidemics overlap in many countries in the developing world. People with HIV are more likely to develop active TB. And HIV-positive people suffering from active TB are three to four times more likely to die than HIV-negative people with TB.

Unlike HIV, which is overwhelmingly transmitted through sexual intercourse, TB is highly contagious. In simple epidemiological terms, the consequences of widespread HIV/TB co-infection are frightening. It is not so much a vicious circle as a vicious spiral: the more cases of active TB there are, the more cases there will be. "It's a simple equation," says Nunn. "More TB means more transmission, and more transmission means more cases [42]." For WHO, the impact of the twin epidemics of HIV and TB on resource-poor countries has "ominous social and medical implications" because "the already over-stretched health services now have to face a tremendously increasing TB problem [43]."

In some African countries it is estimated that up to 60% of TB patients are co-infected with HIV. TB has already become the prime cause of death in adults with HIV in Africa. A recent study in Côte d'Ivoire showed that 35% of adults with HIV died of TB. "TB is the most important HIV-associated disease in Africa," Sebastian Lucas, author of the study, told the VIIIth International Conference on AIDS. "Since Africa has 65% of all cases of HIV, that makes TB the most important AIDS-associated infection in the world."

The devastating potential of this twin epidemic was starkly demonstrated recently when researchers used mathematical models to try to establish its impact on sub-Saharan Africa. In their most optimistic prediction, assuming a low risk of TB infection and low HIV prevalence rates, the researchers calculated that the number of cases of active TB in the 15-49 age group will increase by two-thirds by the turn of the century. Their most pessimistic forecasts suggested a 12-fold increase by the year 2000. The study draws some grim conclusions: "It appears that HIV infection is, as it were, pushing the epidemiological clock back towards the time of the first encounter of human populations with tubercle bacilli." It warns that there is every reason to expect the increase in TB cases to continue well into the twenty-first century [44].

TB chemoprophylaxis—administering anti-TB drugs to HIV-positive people to prevent the onset of active TB—could save thousands, perhaps tens of thousands, of lives and simultaneously help limit the spread of the epidemic. But the cost is enormous. WHO has been conducting a study in Uganda on the feasibility of mass chemoprophylaxis, but "the preliminary results suggest a lot of difficulties [45]".

Despite the gravity of the situation in Africa, doctors and epidemiologists are most anxious about the potential spread of HIV/TB co-infection in Asia where around two-thirds of the world's 1.7 billion TB-infected population is concentrated. Ishwar Gilada, of the Indian Health Association, believes the seeds of a public health disaster have already been sown: "In 1988/89 a survey at a hospital in Bombay found that 2% of TB patients were also infected with HIV. This figure has increased to about 10-15% in the past two years. I have very little hope for the year 2000. India is heading for a major health catastrophe [46]."

Neil McKenna, *adapted from WorldAIDS, September 1992*

The Implications for Hospital Care

Many of the countries now most affected by HIV/AIDS were not able to provide adequate treatment for all cases of curable illnesses, such as malaria, before the epidemic; AIDS is now competing for the same resources.

Within a decade, the pattern of hospital admissions throughout Central Africa has changed radically. A Zaire study reported that 50% of patients at Mama Yemo hospital in Zaire were HIV-positive [27], although not all were being treated for symptoms of AIDS. Twenty-six per cent of patients in the ADZAM hospital study had symptoms resulting from HIV infection (tuberculosis in two-thirds of cases), while a further 12%, treated for injury and other diseases, were HIV-positive [28].

Zaire experts have written: "When one considers that the number of beds at Mama Yemo has not changed over the past 15 years, that it was operating at capacity 15 years ago before there were [any] AIDS cases, and that the population of Kinshasa has been growing rapidly in the interim, it seems that the most important effect of AIDS on the hospital has been to displace one-half of the patients who would otherwise have been treated in the medical wards [29]". One possible further implication of overcrowding is an increase in the number of hospital-acquired infections [30].

In Central Africa, in order to reduce the pressure on hospital beds and staff, there have been successful experiments in alternative methods of care, such as mobile clinics. These alternatives, however, remain extremely rare and are not necessarily cheaper. A preliminary ADZAM costing found that one home-based care visit cost approximately the same as six or seven days in a male medical ward. Since each patient is visited an average of five times before death, the cost of home-based care was equivalent to approximately a month in hospital [31]: $164. (However, this calculation includes the cost of a replacement vehicle, without which the cost could be halved [32].)

Hospitals face more than financial strain. Sister Maura O'Donahue of the UK non-government organisation CAFOD gives the example of a hospital in Uganda with 400 beds and only four doctors, three of whom are relatively inexperienced. "Apart from the increased workload the greatest impact seems to be on the nerves and emotions. Young people are dying, many of them friends of the staff concerned, with consequent greater strain. Staff were accustomed previously to a cure rate of 90% or more. Now that AIDS has entered the scene, the main task of staff

In a decade, the pattern of hospital admissions throughout Central Africa has changed radically

Facing the challenge: a district hospital in Africa

Now that the HIV epidemic is well and truly under way in Southern and Central Africa, patients with AIDS and HIV disease are no longer the subject of medical curiosity, to be prodded and photographed by eminent experts at a central teaching hospital. Instead, patients are increasingly seeking help from their local health services, and every hospital in areas of high infection is having to adapt and adjust.

The biggest impact has been on the staff. In 1991 approximately one employee a month died, out of a total of 300. They included some of the most senior and respected members of staff. The cause is often understood, but not always openly acknowledged, to be AIDS. Other staff are under treatment for HIV disease and the number of deaths will certainly increase over the next few years. Demands to attend the numerous funerals [which can last several days] are especially heavy on the senior staff. Local culture means attending funerals is imperative, but the number has multiplied to such an extent that it has become difficult to staff the hospital adequately, and there is talk of limiting the number of days off for funerals.

Nurses are increasingly worried about occupational exposure, even though research has shown that it is not a significant source of infection. This is little consolation to the nurses, nearly half of whose patients are HIV-positive.

Perhaps surprisingly, the impact of HIV/AIDS on the hospital budget has its positive aspects. Additional funds have been made available for home-based care and counselling, research and training, and have paid for a number of welcome new vehicles and bicycles. But drugs, nursing aids and ward supplies are in as short supply as ever and there is little indication that the needs of AIDS patients have been taken into account in national planning for drug supply.

In particular, drugs for TB are a problem: they are not only costly but are entirely funded by one donor. HIV- positive patients often react, sometimes fatally, to the cheapest anti-TB regimens (based on thiacetazone), and many feel that it has become unethical to use them to treat HIV-positive patients. However, only the cheaper drugs are in sufficient supply and 70%-80% of TB patients are HIV-positive. Doctors are left with a dilemma: to dispense the cheaper drugs and hope patients do not react, or not to treat some TB patients at all. There have already been a number of deaths due to particularly distressing drug reactions, but the problem remains unsolved. Donors have been unwilling to get involved in what they view as a long-term prospect of providing funds for care of HIV disease.

The hospital depends on donations for about 20% of its recurrent budget, especially for AIDS-related activities, and the level of effort required to maintain these donations and report back to the numerous donors is increasing. The hospital is easily accessible from the capital and there is on average one delegation a week requiring the attention of the medical officer in charge, the district medical officer, the hospital administrator and other staff. The district medical officer spends one day in five with visitors and donor representatives, and the hospital administrator spends about a fifth of his time preparing reports and accounts for them. Often visitors must be housed and fed, since the local hotel is not up to international standards. But without these donations, the hospital could not survive, and the quality of care—and staff morale—would suffer tremendously.

Often donors unwittingly create imbalances in hospital activities. For example, the home-based care programme has a vehicle and operating funds, but the TB control officer has no resources to track defaulters from TB treatment—most of whom are HIV-positive.

One solution is for the home-based programme to work with the TB control officer to find out what has happened to people who do not come for follow-up treatment.

Screening blood and indeed finding enough safe blood for transfusion has become a problem. Transfusions are given only in the direst emergencies or when a known safe donor is available. About 20% of potential donors are HIV-positive. The supply of HIV test kits has been erratic and when there is a shortage, screening for transfusions has to take priority. Using them for diagnosis comes second. Using the kits for voluntary testing has to come last, although people are increasingly coming forward to be tested. They want to know their HIV status in order to make important decisions about their lives, such as whether to get married or to have children. But because the hospital cannot cope with the potential demand, voluntary testing remains sporadic and is not actively encouraged.

The hospital is part of the local community and its staff are drawn from it. They have seen many of their neighbours, friends and workmates fall ill and die of AIDS. But since virtually everyone in the district knows someone who has died of AIDS, the stigma appears to be declining. People with HIV/AIDS are not isolated but receive sympathy and understanding. The perception seems to be that AIDS hits almost at random, that anyone could get it. I have never heard of a patient not receiving the best care the hospital could provide, or of a surgeon refusing to operate, or of a nurse shunning a patient because of their HIV status. People here are "facing the challenge" in the most human and humane way possible.

Panos correspondent

members is to help people die with dignity, a task they have not been prepared for [33]." In order to cope with this changing pattern, health personnel need continual education and updating on the disease, and whole new areas of counselling and care need to be introduced or strengthened. In the words of WHO consultant Ndiki Ngcongco: "Nurses...consider themselves crucial to the provision of effective care to HIV/AIDS patients...they are, however, not sufficiently technically competent as they are not equipped with the requisite skills for providing holistic, compassionate and scientific care to HIV/AIDS patients and families. [I forecast] a revolution in AIDS care in Africa—this is nursing's agenda for the 1990s [34]."

An Impossible Burden?

To get some idea of the potential total medical costs of AIDS, figures can be compiled by multiplying the price of individual treatment by the number of those estimated as HIV-positive. There are problems with such figures, however, with some researchers arguing that not everyone with HIV who develops severe symptoms will enter hospital or has access to hospital care. Many others do not do so until the end of their illness: Susan Foster of ADZAM has pointed out that in families in urban areas of Zambia will bring a seriously ill relative to die in hospital,

Ruhengeri hospital, Rwanda

Ruhengeri is Rwanda's fourth largest town, a busy transit centre for the interior, and for Zaire and Uganda. The population of 30,000 had a HIV-positive rate of 21.8% in 1986, the second highest in the country. Since then, the overall rate has not been updated but testing of women attending the antenatal clinic in Ruhengeri hospital from 1989-91 indicated an infection rate of 20.9%, while the rate of those attending the hospital for STDs was 50%.

The number of AIDS cases has been growing at such a rate that it is becoming difficult to hospitalise all the patients. In 1989 the five leading causes of illness in Rwanda were malaria (1,234,099 cases); worms (373,676); respiratory diseases (341,867); broncho-pneumonia (183,385); and diarrhoeal diseases (169,858). Malaria was the main cause of death (1,611 cases), followed by broncho-pneumonia (610), then diarrhoeal diseases (256) and malnutrition (226). Although there were only 960 reported cases of AIDS, it was the fifth leading cause of death (207). By 1990, AIDS had become the third leading cause of death (362), after malaria (2,093) and respiratory diseases (760). There were 2,105 reported cases of AIDS.

Dr Hitimana, who follows up AIDS cases at Ruhengeri hospital, points out that all AIDS statistics are incomplete because not all people with AIDS visit hospital, nor are all those who die of AIDS-related symptoms tested and notified as AIDS deaths. Stigma against AIDS patients, within the hospital as well as the wider community, still exists, so that some patients lack friends or relatives willing to provide the kind of support they need—for example, bringing food soft enough to eat, making the bed, washing clothes and so on. Relations between husband and wife can suffer tremendously when one is discovered to be HIV-positive. Many members of the hospital, from doctors to social workers, themselves lack sufficient knowledge about HIV and AIDS and are consequently ill-prepared to deal with patients. "Many of our nurses do not even want to touch these patients", says Dr Hitimana, "nor do our social workers know exactly what to tell them." This, he adds, makes an AIDS patient a miserable patient who, rather than gaining solace at the hospital, gains more stress.

Patients may try all sorts of cures, explains Dr Hitimana, and visit different doctors and clinics which they cannot really afford—since they have often lost most of their income through being fired or unable to work in the fields. Some are left with no money at all: "In some cases we have to provide coffins and look for workers to dig the grave."

A group of medical staff, charity and social workers, and religious personnel have come together to help raise funds and provide other support for AIDS patients and their relatives, including the growing numbers of orphans. Based at the hospital, the volunteer association visits the families of patients to provide counselling as well as medicines, food, soap and clothing, and help with school fees, book and uniforms. "It is not easy to find something to help everyone with a need," declares Dr Hitimana, president of the association. "But every small thing counts, and people are really beginning to understand about AIDS."

because the cost of transporting a living person there is much less than the cost of transporting a body to the mortuary [35].

Nevertheless, what the figures suggest is that countries face seemingly impossible costs as a result of HIV/AIDS. If predicted treatment costs are multiplied by the estimated number of persons suffering from AIDS in 1990, the potential cost in Tanzania is estimated to amount to 40.6% of the public health budget (and almost 25% of combined public and private spending). In Rwanda, the cost of treating all existing AIDS cases is predicted to equal 65.5% of the public health budget [36]. In South Africa, a medical economist has predicted that 75 billion Rand ($26.8 billion)—10 times the country's 1990 health budget—would be needed to pay for the 1.3 million AIDS cases predicted for 2000. The estimate was based on a figure of R55,000 ($19,650) per patient for an 18-month period between diagnosis and death [37].

The long incubation period means real economic and social costs remain hidden

Meanwhile, actual spending continues to reflect the meagre resources available. Instead of the theoretical 65.5% calculated for Rwanda, the expenditure on all known hospitalised AIDS cases in 1990 was estimated to be $600,000, representing 4.6% of the country's public sector hospital budget. This proportion is predicted to rise to 11.4% by 1994 [38].

In many other countries the overall medical costs of AIDS are not known, with the Zimbabwean response typical of many: "The Ministry of Health currently is not aware of the cost of AIDS cases to the budget. The position is that each case will be treated to the best of the ability of the medical services at whatever level it is seen. It is possible that the patient will be referred up through the system until he reaches the central or general hospitals. It is understood that the Ministry is currently examining these costs and the results of this study should be considered urgently [39]." Without a clearer picture of the real costs involved, it is almost impossible to decide how best to use available resources for AIDS patients, while minimising the diversion of resources from other parts of the health sector.

Clearly, such costs cannot be met unless there is a substantial increase in per capita health expenditure, unlikely in many developing countries which are already struggling to cope, and face further economic decline. In sub-Saharan Africa, an increase in health expenditure would be only a temporary solution. As Anderson's study points out: "Even with substantial injections of financial, physical and human resources it will become increasingly difficult for countries in sub-Saharan Africa to meet the health needs of HIV-positive individuals without compromising the provision of health care to those who are not infected. Decisions have to be made on how scarce health resources should be allocated between prevention and treatment of HIV infection and other diseases [40]."

` Finally, the "impossible costs" of AIDS have to be seen in the

The only feasible long-term solution is a reduction in transmission context of the other impossible costs faced by most developing countries, which are struggling to deal with a whole range of illnesses and other aspects of ill health with health budgets sometimes lower than $5 per head per year. The fact that the choices in HIV/AIDS care are so stark serves to highlight fundamental questions about how poor countries decide priorities and allocate resources about all health issues, not just AIDS.

Care as Prevention

Some health professionals feel that the attention paid to AIDS has led to other health problems being overshadowed, and that resources could be directed to more "cost-effective" purposes than care of HIV/AIDS patients. Diseases such as malaria currently affect far greater numbers of people. Other diseases also claim more lives at present: nearly 13 million children died in 1990, many from easily preventable illnesses. Over 3 million died from diarrhoeal disease and 880,000 died of measles [41].

But none of these diseases has the capacity for relentless growth which AIDS has so far demonstrated. Currently, there is no cure, no vaccine, and treatment is by expensive drugs. Not only is it spread predominantly through one of the most private and sensitive areas of human activity, but its long incubation period means the real economic and social costs remain hidden until the virus has gained a massive hold. These last characteristics make it particularly hard to persuade governments and individuals to take preventive action. Yet, as this chapter has shown, the possible magnitude of the epidemic and its associated medical costs mean that resources are unlikely ever to keep pace with demand. The only feasible long-term solution is a reduction in transmission of the virus. And one of the most effective ways to do this is to couple care with prevention.

Care for AIDS patients is about more than the latest drugs and therapies, or palliation of physical pain and discomfort. It is about psychological support and reassurance and counselling for patients, their families and friends—and this has a knock-on preventive effect for all involved. Prevention messages based on shock and fear have proved to be less effective than education which grows out of understanding and experience: many prejudices have been overcome through direct contact with people with AIDS. So one way of reducing the spread is to build on models of care which feed into prevention activities and so in turn work to reduce the burden of expenditure on health costs. Some ways of doing this are explored in Chapter 8.

CHAPTER 4

Social costs: HIV/AIDS and the community

" "A IDS must be regarded as a community crisis, not simply an individual problem: one which is likely to adversely affect entire communities by threatening their collective ability to cope," states a report on the impact of the epidemic in East and Central Africa [1]. More than any other disease, HIV/AIDS has the potential to undermine both the social and economic fabric of affected communities, because it targets those in the reproductive and "breadwinning" ages, and because its spread is a factor of the way individuals relate to each other. This last characteristic means that the virus has often brought in its wake recrimination and stigma, but above all it implies that "HIV prevention and care requires a cultural sensitivity and community intimacy unparalleled in other health challenges [2]." Thus community responses have emerged from groups of individuals who identify with each other not just on a geographical basis but from common interest, such as the gay (homosexual) community (see Chapter 8 for examples of HIV/AIDS campaigns by such groups).

In a study on sub-Saharan Africa, it was noted that: "Many social systems which are extremely important in the normality of day-to-day life for the largest proportion of African people will be challenged, stressed and possibly changed by the epidemic [3]." While it is vital for policymaking to uncover the potential economic costs of HIV/AIDS, to get a more complete picture of the potential impact of the disease, it is also necessary to consider some of the social institutions and practices which it may affect. For example, if people change their sexual behaviour in order to reduce the threat of HIV/AIDS, how might this affect marriage patterns? What might be the result of so many children being orphaned or brought up by grandparents? How will existing coping mechanisms in the community adapt to the impact of the epidemic? What is the effect on the extended family system? As the disease becomes more widespread, is prejudice increasing or being replaced by compassion and understanding? These are some of the issues explored in this chapter.

In some parts of Africa, HIV/AIDS is known as the "family disease"

The family

Throughout history the family has formed the fundamental social and economic unit on which most human societies have been based. The definition of family varies according to culture and ranges from the single household or nuclear family of parent(s) and child(ren) to a broader kinship network, or extended family, of grandparents, aunts, uncles, cousins and other relatives and individuals. While the status, number and obligations of parents and other adults may vary, such extended households generally function as an economic whole. Although it is usually the adults between the ages of 20 and 50 who bring in the greatest income, all family members may contribute according to their abilities; a child of five can oversee livestock while her 70-year-old grandmother cooks the family meals.

It is not surprising that in some parts of Africa, HIV/AIDS is known as "the family disease". Because the virus predominantly attacks the sexually active, most people who are HIV-positive live in a family with partner and children. The long incubation period of the virus means that even those who contract HIV when single or childless are likely to have formed families by the time they fall ill. Furthermore, because HIV infection is transmitted between couples, and to offspring, there is a strong probability of multiple cases within a household, creating an even greater burden for its members.

Coping Mechanisms

Few developing countries can afford the social welfare systems which the industrialised countries provide for their citizens. More facilities are available in large urban centres but for most people in developing countries, in times of need and crisis it is most often the extended family, whatever its socio-economic status or structure, which is the primary source of support, with secondary assistance provided by friends and neighbours. These coping mechanisms derived from family and social networks limit the impact of ill-health or injury. Colleagues may take on the labour or working responsibilities of the sick person, in the expectation of similar help when they need it. At home, preparation of food, work on the land or looking after livestock will be done by another family member or neighbour in addition to their own tasks.

The longer an individual is incapacitated, the more likely it is that the loss of their labour will have an economic impact. The person who takes on their work may do so at the expense of other productive activities. Long-term investment in education, for

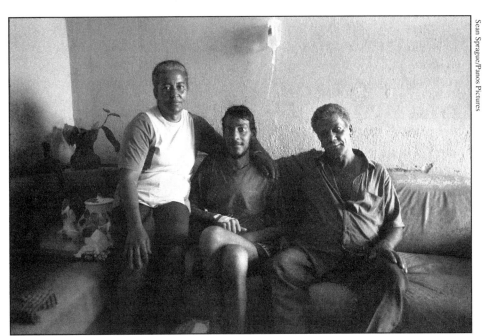

Families are the first to take the strain of caring for someone with HIV/AIDS, like the parents of this 27-year-old Brazilian. As the number of affected families increases, the coping mechanisms of the wider community are put under pressure.

example, may be affected by taking children away from school to compensate or care for an ill adult. The need to buy medicines or special foods may eat into the budget for other food, household necessities or farm equipment. Savings may be reduced and assets sold. Death leads to expenditure on mourning ceremonies and may be followed by changes in the composition of the household, as children are fostered and/or the surviving spouse moves away or remarries.

The effect of HIV/AIDS operates at three different levels: the individual, the family and the wider society. And in any community, the greater the number of households affected by a disease such as HIV/AIDS, the greater the strain on wider social coping systems. More families, more frequently, find themselves asked to contribute to the funeral expenses of neighbours and relatives, to assist in financing health care, to take on work in their fields, care for the sick or take in orphaned children. The arrival of two, three and often more orphans from other parts of the extended family obviously has dramatic effects on the survival strategies of rural households which are already under stress, although older children will be able to contribute extra labour and in some cases their parents' land.

Over time, the ability of family and social networks to absorb these demands decreases. Researchers have found that coping mechanisms in Uganda are being extended to such an extent that

*Most
communities
go through
three stages:
denial,
acceptance,
then action*

solutions previously considered unusual are now being utilised. For instance, if there is no-one to look after a man's children after his death, "women who have severed relationships with the deceased man, either through desertion or divorce...may now reappear on his death to look after his children from a later relationship [4]."

In many rural areas, families depend heavily on the earnings of one or more members who have migrated to find work. If the migrant worker falls ill and returns home, families face a double burden of having to compensate for lost income and also care for the sick person.

The situation in urban areas is not much better. A study led by Maxine Ankrah of Uganda's Makerere University came to the conclusion that HIV/AIDS is producing a crisis in urban family maintenance and functioning that the extended family cannot address. The study identified five areas of need created by HIV/AIDS. These comprised basic food and housing plus income or economic assistance; medical care; accurate information and health education; HIV testing opportunities for spouses/regular partners; and psychological and social support [5].

City dwellers and their families tend to be more isolated than do those in more close-knit, rural communities. It may follow from this that urban residents are more autonomous, economically and socially, and less dependent on each other than are their rural counterparts, with the possible advantage that the secondary impact when somebody dies will be lower. A disadvantage is that extended family and community support systems are also likely to be weaker in urban areas, with the result that when individuals need that kind of support they tend to return to their home village.

Stages of response

HIV/AIDS brings more than medical and economic problems. The stigma still associated with the disease in many communities may mean some people are less willing to help individuals and families; it also increases the emotional burden on people with HIV/AIDS and their carers. Ankrah's study confirmed that some people whose parents or children had died from AIDS but who had not themselves contracted HIV, were nevertheless stigmatised, which interfered with their ability to recover from the emotional and financial consequences of the disease.

However, as more individuals and households within a community are directly affected by the disease, experience suggests that discrimination can give way to greater understanding and willingness to give support. One report on community responses identifies three broad stages, which are related to the level of infection within a community. In the initial stage, when cases are few, reactions are characterised by fear, despair and "barely concealed panic" about preventing further spread of the disease. This is when ostracism of people with AIDS and their families is most likely. As the number of cases grows and more people are themselves infected and affected by the death of partners and relatives, there is greater concern to find ways of coping both with people with AIDS and with their dependants. If counselling is available, this can do much to change rejection to acceptance and to help get "people back into an active frame of mind to work together to help themselves and also others".

Outside assistance should go towards strengthening existing community mechanisms and initiatives

In the third and final stage, "when death is commonplace", the crisis is seen as one affecting everyone, not just individual groups or families. Communities tend to function more cohesively, building on existing support systems or developing new ones: "Care of the dying becomes an important focus with the development of home-care, hospices and support systems for those dying and bereaved [6]."

The extent to which a community can survive this third phase, however, obviously reflects the resources available; some may "simply collapse under the strain of supporting a large proportion of ill people and bereaved dependants on very limited resources [7]". Since the poorer people in poorer countries have the least access to any government support or welfare systems, this certainly suggests that any outside assistance should go towards strengthening existing community mechanisms and initiatives, and preventing such a collapse. An example of this is the assistance given by Concern, an Irish non-government organisation working in Uganda, to Munno Mukabi, a women's organisation whose members voluntarily give practical and emotional support to people affected by HIV/AIDS (see p102).

Adapting Social Practices

ACORD, another development agency working in East Africa, has noted how existing support groups are beginning to alter certain practices or develop new ones in response to the epidemic. In Uganda, ACORD staff have seen the emergence of new types of burial groups, the traditional purpose of which is to help with funeral costs on a one-off basis. The cost of burial and funeral ceremonies can be very high, involving several days of mourning during which work ceases for all participants and many relatives

A community fights back

Even if 35-year-old Ham Katongole, of Rakai district in southwest Uganda, had not put into words how HIV/AIDS had devastated his home region, his rugged miserable face vividly tells all. "Most of us here have given up on life. During the past five years, I have lost 14 of my children and their mother," he said, pointing at the row of mud-filled graves in the courtyard of his tin-roofed house.

"We are always busy burying the dead in this village and have no time left to work in the gardens. The small savings we have, we spend on the sick and when they die, they leave us poor and we have to look after the orphans."

A report carried out in five villages in Rakai by the Psychology Department at Makerere University found evidence of depression being experienced on a massive scale [42]. It manifests itself in poor communication within families, between individuals, and between community leaders and members. There is lack of cohesion in the community, and traditional groupings for mutual help and support, such as the extended family system, are collapsing. Juvenile delinquency among unemployed youth is on the increase. In addition to the depression caused by widespread bereavement and increasing poverty, there are accusations and counter accusations among the men, women and younger people as to who is mainly responsible for spreading the disease.

The report found that many men drink heavily to relieve their depression, sorrow and worries. Brewing is one of the few economic opportunities open to widows, whose husbands have often died of AIDS. After drinking, some of these men sleep with the widows. Some become infected with HIV and then transmit the disease to their wives. This leads to more sickness and death, which is the main cause of their depression. "As a result, men in Rakai district are trapped in a vicious circle of poverty, booze and AIDS," concludes the study. The men of Rakai have been unable to break out of this vicious circle because there is no definite place where people can go and get help; and there are few organised groups to advise people, many of whom are reluctant to share their problems.

Researchers say that poverty is rife in Rakai villages, as elsewhere in rural Uganda, because prices of the agricultural commodities on which they depend for income are low, while manufactured goods are expensive. All this is exacerbated in areas badly affected by HIV/AIDS because of low productivity, in turn caused by constant HIV-related illness, as well as time spent nursing the sick and attending the daily round of funerals.

According to the study, although farming was the most important activity in Rakai about four years ago—occupying 98% of the local people—the majority of men (61.7%) are now engaged in petty trade. Traditionally, men were expected to grow the cash crops, such as coffee and bananas. They also planted vegetables like cabbages and tomatoes. Similarly, some 60% of the women—traditionally responsible for growing all the food for the household—are now engaged in business and animal husbandry. Part of the reason for the change is economic—the poor return for farming produce—but much of the change in occupation reflects loss of labour for cultivation, which meant some farms were no longer viable. It also reflects the need by those who are ill to find work which takes less physical energy.

Women are now engaged in petty trade and selling secondhand clothes, as well as making handicrafts, keeping poultry and rearing pigs. These activities help them to pay school fees for their children and for other basic necessities. They are less time-consuming than farmwork, and so enable women to look after sick children and relatives, for which they

take much more responsibility than men.
Some men have abandoned their support of the household because the women are now engaged in money-generating activities and can partly support their families. Some resent the women's income and claim they no longer have full control over their wives because they do not stay in the villages but travel to towns and markets to carry out their business. Some husbands are jealous of their womenfolk because of the differences in their income. Although the traditional tribal brotherhood groups have broken down as villages have collapsed under the social and economic strain of HIV/AIDS, some men are now forming cooperative societies, such as the Kapapali Cooperative Society for brewers of alcohol, cultivators and builders. But the intensity of the poverty is such that it is hard to raise enough capital. In addition, they need training in how to run a cooperative. Women's coping mechanisms have been rather more successful, and they have formed several mutual help societies which provide support to the ill and the bereaved but also generate funds through, for example, group cultivation and small investments in other income generating schemes.
The local people, building on help from non-government organisations (NGOs) such as Concern, an Irish NGO, have now decided to work together and to revive some traditional community organisations; to provide orphans with education and vocational training (for example, in brickmaking and carpentry); to involve the whole community in economic projects; and to increase their self-reliance by getting training in project management. There is also a move to make more use of available resources, such as locally grown dyes (*muzuukizi*) in their handicrafts. Concern has been helping people diversify from farming, providing training in accounts and cooperative management. They have supported the women's income-generating schemes and given them training in health care.
All these are encouraging signs that people are prepared to work together and fight the effects of HIV/AIDS. Clearly, in the 10 years since the virus was first diagnosed in the region, which was already suffering from the traumatic years of civil war, village societies have come close to collapse, but the community spirit is still there and with support new or revived coping mechanisms are beginning to emerge.
David Musoke, *Rakai*

and friends must be fed and housed by the family concerned. In areas where many people are dying from HIV/AIDS, there is anecdotal evidence that much working time is being lost through funeral attendance. Communities are making changes, however. Whereas three-day wakes used to be common, ACORD staff have noticed that in badly affected areas, funeral ceremonies are getting shorter and therefore less costly in time and money.

This observation is backed up by a study in Rakai, Uganda: "Bodies are usually buried within a day or two of death, which allows little time for kin to come from a distance to funerals and mourning ceremonies....They mostly take place in the early evening and several might be attended in one evening at neighbouring homesteads [8]." The new burial groups are more permanent, better structured, and work collectively—fishing,

Some village leaders have suggested reducing bridewealth to slow the spread of AIDS

cultivating, selling produce or timber—to raise funds to lend to widows for medical and other expenses, in addition to funeral costs. Some have developed self-financed credit schemes. ACORD is supporting these groups and exploring their potential for developing a wider social welfare function.

Other documented examples of modifications to existing social customs include the banning of certain types of traditional dances, and the discouragement of in-laws from "inheriting" their brothers' widows. Traditional healers, who are often responsible for, among other things, circumcision and scarification, are requesting that customers and patients bring their own knives or razor blades rather than re-using their own instrument. ACORD is exploring the possibility of traditional healers and herbalists, who are now forming their own associations, developing an active counselling and educational role [9].

Patterns of marriage may undergo some changes because of HIV/AIDS. In Uganda, according to one study, some village leaders have "suggested reducing bridewealth and eliminating levirate [the custom of compulsory marriage with a childless brother's widow] to prevent or slow the spread of AIDS". Because it takes time to accumulate the necessary resources, "high bridewealth is thought to delay marriage, increasing the prospective groom's likelihood of using commercial sex workers while he waits. Levirate can spread the virus through an entire extended family [10]."

Some researchers predict there may be a substantial reduction of extramarital relations and an earlier age of male marriage. For women, increased education and autonomy should mean the age of marriage going up, but the public response to HIV/AIDS may reverse such gains [11]. The practice of men seeking younger female partners on the basis that they are less likely to be infected has already been noted. There may also be more widows, since women in particular find it hard to remarry after their spouse has died of AIDS, because they are suspected of having given the disease to their partner.

The effect on attitudes to fertility is as yet unclear. Certainly, the desire to conceive precludes sex with a condom, and for many women the social stigma of being childless may outweigh the risk of becoming infected. One response to large numbers of deaths in a community may be a rise in births, as parents seek to compensate for the toll of AIDS, but there are as yet no detailed studies on this.

One aspect of community life which may be affected is

support and exchange systems such as communal labour groups, based on reciprocation. If more and more families become unable to meet their social obligations to help others in their fields, will this mean that they will cease to get help themselves at key periods such as planting and harvest time? The situation is exacerbated by the fact that AIDS is regarded as a fatal disease and so such obligations, once suspended, are unlikely to be resumed at a later stage. If such systems break down, there are obvious implications for agricultural productivity.

Women are more likely than men to be driven into destitution in the last days of their life

This picture of a possible breakdown in certain community structures must be tempered with the earlier evidence of the way communities have responded positively, developing new support mechanisms or adapting old ones. In the words of Chandra Mouli, a doctor who has many years' experience of working with communities, especially in Zambia, on HIV/AIDS issues: "AIDS has generated such a strong community response in Africa because it is perceived as everybody's problem. In many countries in sub-Saharan Africa, most people know of a family member, friend or workmate who has died of AIDS. This is a strong motivating force for individual behaviour change and for community action [12]."

Women Bear the Brunt

There are a number of ways in which women are disproportionately affected by the epidemic. As Chapter 1 outlined, the social and economic status of many women makes them less able to protect themselves from infection. If infected, they face the prospect of passing on the disease to any children they may bear. They also take on a greater share of the burden of caring for the sick. And when they themselves fall ill, they face more problems than men. Some husbands reject their wives, even though they are the source of the women's infection. The Tanzanian community-based AIDS organisation WAMATA reports that women with AIDS are more likely to have to return to their families or place of origin for terminal care, while men are likely to be cared for in their own home. A man continues to be head of household till his death, while a woman gives up that status when she moves out of her home.

Many women lose their rights to certain family assets, including land, when a male relative such as husband or father dies. Women are therefore more likely than men to be driven into destitution in the last days of their life [13]. The sexual nature of HIV transmission means that two of the limited range of

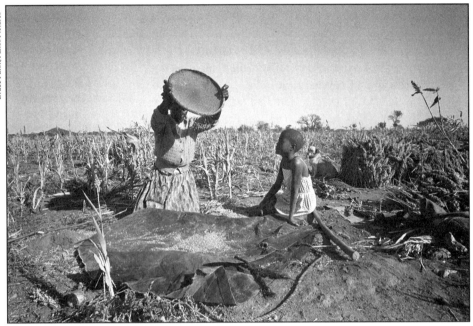

Bruce Paton/Panos Pictures

Cleaning sorghum, Botswana. In many parts of Africa, there is an increasing number of small farms headed by women. Often the poorest of the poor, these households are especially vulnerable to the impact of HIV/AIDS.

economic opportunities open to widows—remarriage within the husband's family, and prostitution—impose serious social costs in the form of disease transmission.

WAMATA also points out that poorer households tend to have a smaller network of support to draw upon in times of need and therefore receive less assistance and fewer contributions of food or other items in comparison with households which have a wide social and professional network [14]. And the poorest of poor households tend to be those headed by women. In particular, small farms headed by women, in their own right or in their husbands' absence, are often in a precarious situation and are already very vulnerable to external blows such as drought, pests, or crop diseases.

Women whose husbands are migrant workers depend heavily on their remittances to pay for the extra labour needed on the farm and to supplement the family's income. The death of their husband not only stops the flow of cash, but also the seasonal labour the men provided themselves and the hired labour they paid for, with a resultant fall in productivity. The number of households headed by women is considerable and on the increase: in Malawi, for example, 33% of farms are headed by women, a figure which rises to 45% in the south of the country [15]. Households are also especially vulnerable where there is severe social control on women, as in Bangladesh, which increases their dependence on the male breadwinner. When the breadwinner is ill or dies, the employment opportunities for women are extremely restricted. Widows without adult sons are particularly likely to become destitute. A study of a poor urban area of Bangladesh found that the risk of malnutrition of all members of households with an incapacitated earner was 2.5 times greater than in households where the male head was working [16].

Inheritance practices have taken on a new importance

When their husbands die, many women find themselves dispossessed of their home and land since the rights to certain assets, including agricultural tools, livestock and property tenancy and ownership, are often vested in men. Referring to sub-Saharan Africa, but making points that are often applicable elsewhere, a UNICEF report argues that: "Inheritance laws and customs also influence women's economic status and even their choice of formal or informal unions in regions where inheritance does not offer women financial protection. In Congo, for example, many women choose not to legalise their relationships, recognizing that any financial assets or property earned with a husband are likely to revert to [him] or their children in the case of death or divorce [17]".

Inheritance practices have taken on a new importance for the increasing numbers of women whose husbands have died of AIDS, and for their orphaned children in cases where the latter were legally not entitled to inheritance, or where relatives take over the property. Tanzania has recently changed inheritance laws to better protect widows [18]. However, the degree to which any laws protect women and children will depend on women's knowledge of and effective access to the legal system [19]. One of ACORD's activities in Uganda is to liaise with Ugandan Women Lawyers (FIDA) and organise a legal awareness programme, mainly to help widows and orphans cope with inheritance issues.

Caring for the sick

Whether at home or in hospital, patient care involves women more than men. A survey by WAMATA found that women both provided more care (more than twice as much as men) and received less care as patients [20].

Where hospitals provide only essential medical treatment, and food and general nursing care must be provided by the patient's family—which is common practice in many developing countries —an added burden is placed on the household and the care giver, especially if the hospital is far from the patient's home. In parts of rural sub-Saharan Africa, the community often supports a

Caring: the cost to a community

"Jona" left Kenya for higher studies abroad when he was 20. His mother, who had two other children at school and college, struggled to find the 30,000 Kenyan shillings (about $1,400) required initially. Unable to raise this sum of money on her own, she organised a *harambee*, whereby the community come together to contribute voluntarily to a worthy cause.

Jona returned home in May 1988, HIV-positive and suffering from oral thrush, diarrhoea, vomiting and loss of more than 10% of his normal body weight. He was in hospital for a total of 14 days. His mother took 90 days' compassionate leave to look after her son; after he passed away she felt she needed time to learn how to "face the world again" because of his loss and to reconcile herself to the fact that he had died of AIDS, a stigmatising disease. The three months were lost work time to the labour force, with economic costs for her employers. One of Jona's brothers also took four weeks' compassionate leave. A sister missed four weeks of high school.

I taught his mother simple nursing techniques. She also required counselling weekly for one month, fortnightly for another month, and two more monthly sessions. If this service had been charged for, it would have been a further financial drain on the family: a supportive and free counselling network is urgently needed to help both rural and urban families cope.

Jona's appetite was poor and he would be choosy about food and drink. So fruits and fruit juice were made abundantly available for him, whereas ordinarily such things were only for special occasions. His mother had a lot of extra expenses.

In Kenya, as in many parts of Africa, we still enjoy the extended family kinship system. On average, 10 people from the village, including distant family members, visited Jona daily. This was to register their solidarity and concern that AIDS had struck their village. Each would visit for an average of one hour. This tremendous social support had, however, an economic cost: 10 working hours lost every day.

Jona was a brave, delightful young man. Nevertheless, he went through all the stages of terminal illness: denial, anger, bargaining, depression and acceptance. He died at peace with himself and the world.

In 1989, "Gregory", a 26-year-old from Bukoba in Tanzania, went to the former Soviet Union for further studies. After a year, he started having bouts of diarrhoea and lost weight steadily. He was found to be HIV-positive and returned to his rural home in late 1990.

One of Gregory's major worries was how to deal with his parents, who had already started traditional mourning. Every evening, and sometimes during the day, villagers came to his home to mourn, at the encouragement of his parents. Living in a patriarchal society, they were deeply ashamed and disappointed that their only son had AIDS and that their investment for their old age had been demolished. This was why they mourned while Gregory was still alive.

Many working hours of the household were used up, as were the working hours of other households in the community. Visitors were offered tea and sometimes food, which led to an additional expense of $15 per month for Gregory's parents—a sum which they could not afford.

Elizabeth Ngugi, *Department of Community Health, University of Nairobi*

patient's family with donations of money, food, fuelwood and other material supplies for supplementary hospital care. Hospital visits may be organised in such a way that there is a regular flow of people taking supplies to the patient and reporting back on their progress to the community.

The ADZAM study of the economic impact of illness in Zambia has examined the cost of "helpers": relatives or friends who visit or stay near the hospital to provide food and care for the patient. Sixty per cent of the study's patient sample had helpers: 74% of these were women, with an average age of 42, half of whom gave their occupation as farming. An analysis of costs was not available at the time of publication, but it is significant that in answer to the question, "What is the biggest problem facing you now?" 36% of helpers replied that it was provision of food [21].

There is a strong correlation between parental mortality and the mortality of children under 10

The price children pay
High birth rates in many countries severely affected by HIV/AIDS means that the number of children infected and affected by the disease is also high. Whatever the cause, children are likely to be seriously affected by the illness or death of their parents. Research in Bangladesh, quoted in a World Bank study, pointed to a strong correlation between parental mortality and the mortality of children under 10 years old. A father's death was associated with an increase of 6 per 1,000 in the child mortality rate. A mother's death was associated with an increase of almost 50 per 1,000 deaths for sons and 144 per 1,000 for daughters, compared to rates of 27 per 1,000 for boys and 42 per 1,000 for daughters with no parental death.

The World Bank study points out some reasons why: "The household's attempt to cope with the death or ill-health of an adult may shift household labor away from health maintaining activities such as cleaning, collecting water, hygienic food preparation and breast-feeding." There is a greater likelihood of malnutrition if a brother or sister or grandparent has to look after the children. In a study of the nutritional status of the young children of Filipino working mothers, 55% of children younger than 36 months who were cared for by siblings (aged six to eight years) were malnourished compared to only 8.5% who were cared for by their mothers. Grandparents and other elderly people were more effective care givers than siblings, but still induced malnutrition in 21% of the young children [22]. These findings are especially relevant to HIV/AIDS because uninfected children born to HIV-positive mothers are often already underweight and

Orphans

The increasing number of adult deaths from HIV/AIDS in Central Africa leaves more and more children orphaned (lacking one or both parents). UNICEF predicts that there will be 3-5 million orphans in 10 Central and East African countries by the end of the century, more than half of which will be in rural communities; the higher figure represents more than 1 in 10 of all children under 15 [33]. Timothy Stamps, Zimbabwe Minister of Health, predicts that of every 1,000 children born there, 140 will be orphaned by the age of 10 [34]. In Thailand, 2 million children are expected to be motherless by 2010 [35].

Most other diseases and epidemics claim the very young and the elderly, rarely both parents of young children as HIV/AIDS does. Traditionally, orphans in Africa are taken in by members of the extended family, but this is becoming less feasible in areas with many AIDS deaths. More and more, parentless children find themselves living with grandparents, in institutions—or homeless.

Children orphaned by HIV/AIDS face many social and psychological problems, as highlighted by James Ssekiwanuka of the Save the Children Fund in Uganda. Orphans lose out economically: when their sick parents use up all the family resources to pay for medical care, or when relatives take their land because they themselves cannot look after it. If taken in by the extended family, their living conditions and diet are likely to be poor. This, together with lack of immunisation and health care, heightens their vulnerability to disease. Their status—in itself a stigma—reduces their chances of marriage. If not taken in by relatives, they may become "street children", and highly vulnerable to HIV/AIDS because of the need to sell sexual favours for cash or food, or they may end up being institutionalised, which creates other problems of adapting to society [36].

Another Ugandan study, which traced 460 5-15-year-olds, children of 150 people who had died of AIDS, found high levels of deprivation. Seventy per cent had neither mother nor father. More than one in three had been abandoned or were in institutions; almost two in three had left school as result of lack of fees; more than two in three were "virtually naked" and malnourished; one in 30 had been sexually abused; and two in five showed signs of psychological disorder. James Lwanga, author of the study, noted that: "Children are abandoned and stigmatised by relatives, friends and society at large. They suffer psychologically and their rights [are] abused." Lwanga goes on to argue for the need to create supportive environments, offering counselling, psychological and material support for these children [37].

less healthy than babies born to HIV-negative mothers.

Although unlikely to be infected, older children are also affected by the epidemic. They may find themselves caring for sick parents rather than being cared for themselves. The death of parents leaves many families headed by 14- or 15-year-olds, who must take on the role of family providers. Like their mothers, their rights to land owned or leased by their family are jeopardised by a father's early death [23]. If the household breaks up and the children go to live with relatives or enter a new environment, they may undergo considerable stress. Apart from having to come to terms with their parents' death, they may worry whether they

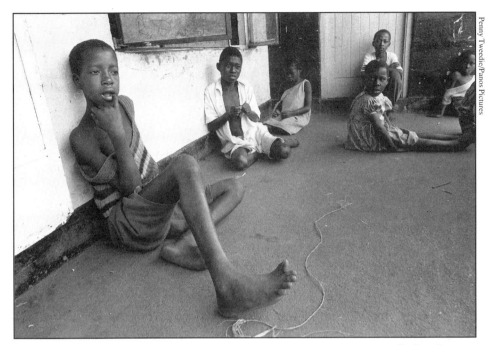

Penny Tweedie/Panos Pictures

Orphans in Uganda. The number of children orphaned by HIV/AIDS in parts of Africa is outstripping the traditional ability of families and communities to care for them.

themselves are infected. Grandparents may be overprotective, and so reduce a child's self-confidence. The children's education may have been interrupted and their concentration is also likely to suffer. Overall, because children have fewer financial, physical and mental resources, the burden of adult illness and death is far greater on them than vice versa [24].

Orphaned children in particular face a number of difficulties. However, a point made by ACORD staff in Uganda is that Northern-based NGOs sometimes see the problem of orphans in isolation and fail to see that they are still part of a community. While this is an area of care and support which has received more attention than most, any programmes to improve the position of orphans have to be culturally sensitive and promote their re-integration into existing families where possible, or support existing community mechanisms [25].

Education

The development aspirations of most countries depend upon increasing levels of education and literacy. Yet in the worst-hit communities, HIV/AIDS is already having an adverse impact on education.

Many families affected by the epidemic cannot afford to keep children in school, because reduced income may mean that

Education: changes in supply and demand

The impact of HIV/AIDS on education can be profound, and has both immediate and long-term effects. Sickness or death of family members—or of children themselves —takes pupils away from school. Yet these institutions could play a considerably bigger part in teaching children—and the local community—how to look after themselves, and how to help prevent the further spread of HIV/AIDS.

The most immediate impact of the epidemic is to reduce demand for education. Fewer children will be born in a society where AIDS is present than if it were not, and most children infected perinatally will develop AIDS and die before reaching school age. Both of these factors will have considerable effect on initial school enrolment. The few children who reach school age with HIV/AIDS may not have the physical strength to enter or continue in school. Also, families will have more need for child labour and less money available for fees and the other indirect costs of schooling. Those orphaned may suffer ostracism, anxiety about their HIV/AIDS status, abandonment or exploitation; their educational motivation will suffer and many will end up as street children. The demand for education for girls may suffer most. "When resources are scarce, the preference for sending boys to school might be strengthened [38]", both because girls' labour is needed in larger households and because they may marry earlier as the pool of older, eligible women decreases due to illness and death, and as men seek younger, uninfected spouses.

Thus, while demand for pre-school and early childhood care may increase, as traditional childminders such as grandparents and older children (re)enter the productive labour force, the demand for primary and secondary school places will probably decrease. One worst case scenario for Tanzania predicts that in 2020, because the school cohort will be smaller when AIDS is present, there will be 22% fewer children to be educated at primary level and 14% fewer at secondary level [39]: this percentage might be considerably higher because of low enrolment and high drop-out rates due to economic and health reasons. Weak demand at these levels of the system will affect demand at the tertiary level. Higher education will also be affected by the illness and death of students who, as sexually active young adults, are prime targets of the disease. Their loss amounts to a loss of trained human resources and of the investment made in them by their families and the education system. Demand for higher education overseas may also fall, as the number of possible candidates decreases, and as sponsors and receiving nations test for HIV. One major provider of overseas fellowships has noticed an increasing number of candidates rejected by its immigration office "for medical reasons" (presumably HIV) and is planning to encourage longer lists of alternative candidates. It has also expressed concern over how much funding can be provided in the country of study for medical treatment and/or repatriation of students with AIDS [40].

The impact on supply of educational places and institutions and of people to fill them is also potentially significant. Educators are among the best trained people in many rural districts and are often influential agents for development even in more cosmopolitan areas. Their numbers will decrease as the cadre of young, better-trained teachers, lecturers, trainers, administrators and planners become ill, are absent from work, and die. Again a scenario in Africa predicts as a worst case, a loss of 27,000 primary school teachers by 2020 [41]. This, coupled with fewer pupils and a smaller base of local financial support from larger families and from economically weakened communities, may eventually lead to ever smaller and finally unviable and abandoned schools.

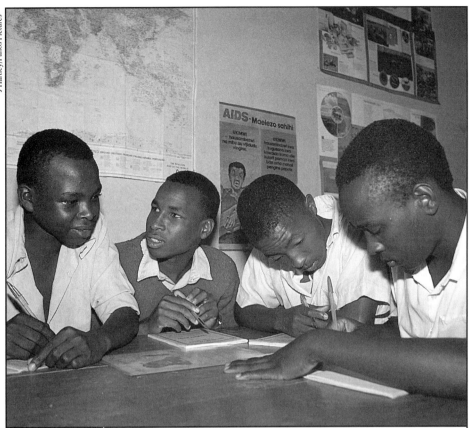

J Hartley/Panos Pictures

Secondary school in Kenya. In the worst-affected areas, HIV/AIDS will reduce the demand for school places and may cause some schools to close down. Yet schools have a vital role to play in reducing the spread and the impact of the disease by becoming centres of education, training and support.

More subtle and ultimately more difficult to confront, is the impact of HIV/AIDS on the process of education. As and when various kinds of formal discrimination and informal harassment of pupils with HIV/AIDS emerge, the impact on the teaching-learning process and on relationships between pupils and teaching staff may be significant.

Over the long term, education systems heavily affected by HIV/AIDS will need to broaden their objectives and functions in order to respond more effectively to the populations they serve. Growing numbers of children may not be enrolled in school: some may be orphaned, psychologically scarred and physically abandoned; others may be members of larger, poorer families unable to afford fees and other expenses, and more likely to be working. To cater for such children, schools will need to be able to provide cheaper and less formal educational programmes, aimed at a wider age range and with more flexible hours. They will need to provide more systematic counselling, both psychological and occupational, and more practical training, in agriculture and home economics for example. And as one of the few institutions found even in quite poor and remote areas, schools will find it necessary to provide a wider range of services, such as literacy courses, child care and health advice, to non-enrolled orphans and other members of the community.

Sheldon Shaeffer, *International Institute for Educational Planning, Paris*

Demand for primary and secondary school places will probably decrease

finding even small amounts of money for fees, uniforms, books or other items is no longer possible. Even where there is no question of school fees, children may be needed at home to look after sick parents or to do their work. This has a cumulative effect, as the longer children stay away from school, the less likely they are to return. Homeless orphans are unlikely to attend school, while grandparents may not have the resources or authority to enable children in their care to continue their education. A 1989 study by the UK non-government organisation Save the Children Fund found that 34% of children were not attending school in the badly affected Rakai region of Uganda [26].

Sheldon Shaeffer of the International Institute for Educational Planning, sees possible shifts in the way schools function and the subjects they offer, reflecting the changing needs of children and their families: "Girls in particular will need new skills to make them financially independent." Shaeffer says that ministries of education will have to become proactive, not only in teaching the basic facts of HIV/AIDS but also on deciding "when to close schools and what, if anything, to replace them with; when and how to recruit and rapidly train new, and often less well-educated, teachers and to perhaps convince them to teach in heavily affected regions; and how to predict more accurately the staffing needs of seriously affected sectors of the economy and then train more people to fill those needs [27]."

The need for action
Initially, the first people to suffer from HIV/AIDS in rural communities were those who travelled a great deal and those who had contact with them (truck drivers and their partners, for example), and the more skilled and educated (village leaders, traders, extension workers) because they were the most likely to visit the urban areas where infection rates are higher. But once the virus enters a community, all kinds of households may be at risk. Relative wealth may allow some families to cope in the short term, but over time the effect of the epidemic will be to increase poverty at a family and community level. The impact of the disease will be prolonged and cumulative, and in many rural areas may lead to long-term problems of nourishment and food security (see Chapter 6).

Studies in Uganda stress the interdependence of the households within communities [28]. Larger, wealthier families employ poorer relatives, help with funerals, hire labour, provide money for school fees and health care. If the whole community is impoverished this coping mechanism will not exist. If steps can

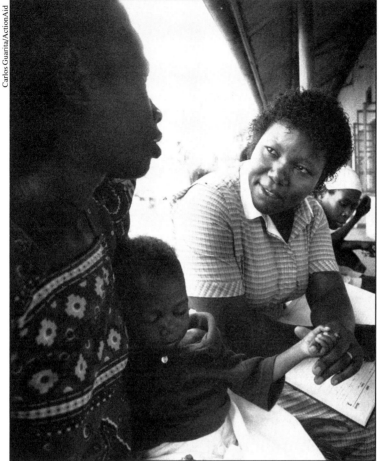

The AIDS Support Organization (TASO) was the first community-based response to the epidemic in Uganda. Since 1987, it has provided thousands of people with information, care and support. Here founding director Noerine Kaleeba counsels a mother at a TASO clinic.

be taken to prevent the spread of the infection or to intervene before community resources are stretched to breaking point, these measures will be much more effective.

Yet because of the long incubation period of the virus, HIV is likely to be well established in a population before the warning signs can no longer be ignored. As experience in Central Africa has shown, coping mechanisms can soon become overwhelmed and the costs of dealing with the impact are already huge by the time it is recognised [29]. Community-based programmes in other regions therefore face the difficult task of addressing the problem before it has become apparent to the population it will affect. Given that most communities seem to go through the three stages of denial, reluctant acceptance and action when faced with HIV/AIDS, the challenge is to cut out denial and complacency and go straight into concerted action.

"HIV is never the number one concern"

"AIDS, unlike people, is not prejudiced," says Toni Phifer. "It doesn't matter what colour your skin is." Phifer knows this all too well. The 31-year-old mother of two is black, and both she and her husband have AIDS. As if having the disease itself was not enough, the couple recently lost their three-year-old daughter, Nia, who was born HIV-positive.

Phifer and her husband are but two of Baltimore's 1,671 African Americans diagnosed with AIDS by April 1992. The Phifers represent a fraction of the estimated 8,000-16,000 HIV-positive among Baltimore's 435,768 African Americans. Blacks account for 79% of Baltimore's AIDS cases, and almost all the city's HIV-positive women and babies are black. Statistically, AIDS has surpassed homicide, heart disease, cancer and accidents as the leading cause of death among Baltimore's 25-44-year-olds. In practice, however, HIV/AIDS takes a back seat to other concerns of poor people, who daily confront more pressing matters.

The Phifers were relatively well off: Toni was an executive secretary and her husband was an accountant. Now she is dependent on social services to supply the 18 different drugs she must take, and to pay the huge medical bills she and her husband have accrued so far this year. But well over a third of the city's black households have annual incomes below the poverty level, defined in 1990 as $13,359. This compares with an average for the state of Maryland of $39,385, the fourth richest in the United States. Some 53,000 black households are headed by a single mother; nearly 14,000 more than two-parent households. Forty-three per cent of the city's black population have never completed high school, compared to a national average of 24%. Only 5.3% have earned bachelor's degrees; the national average is 13%.

Faced with figures such as these, it is no wonder that "HIV is never the number one concern", points out Baltimore City AIDS coordinator Brenda Pridgen. Fear of HIV infection in the black community, she adds, ranks far behind concerns about violence, housing, food, getting to work for those who have a job, or getting the daily fix for those on drugs. "How could HIV be the first concern?" asks Dion Thompson, a reporter for the *Baltimore Sun*, who has spent several months following the efforts of the city's black community churches to address AIDS. "HIV doesn't have the same immediacy," he says. "HIV is just one more thing they have to deal with."

Joe O'Neil, a volunteer doctor at Johns Hopkins University's Moore Clinic, agrees, pointing out that HIV is "often not my patients' leading concern". At the clinic, which sees 1,200 HIV patients, 90% of whom are black, O'Neil says patients are more concerned about the drugs and violence in their neighbourhoods than about their own illness. "Two women patients have had children murdered since I've been caring for them," he adds. As Larry Simmons, ethnic outreach coordinator for the Maryland State AIDS Administration, puts it: "People are listening, but there is still the feeling that 'it's too bad it's happening, but I don't feel it will happen to me'."

Ignorance is not bliss, as a study of STD patients at Johns Hopkins University shows [43]. The 17,207 blood samples taken from the city's STD clinics between 1979 and 1989 (95% from blacks) showed that the rate of HIV infection over the decade had increased from 0.23% to 5.35%. Furthermore, the ratio of HIV-infected men to women is now about even.

For poor African Americans, illness is not considered "serious" unless there are visible, debilitating symptoms, according to Pridgen. This is largely why "historically, for most blacks, primary health care services began in the emergency room," says David H Shippee, director of one of Baltimore's largest AIDS service organisations, about two-thirds of whose clients are black.

Dealing with the present, and doing whatever has to be done to make ends meet, is something Yvonne Veney hears a lot about in the jail where she provides HIV prevention education to women, 95% of whom are black. It may mean risking HIV infection from sex with a promiscuous and/or drug-injecting male partner, but if he brings money into the house, Veney says, a woman will not insist he uses a condom. She explains: "The possibility of having food and a house for a child outweighs the probability of getting infected....This is why you can't do [HIV education] in a vacuum."

Misinformation and denial of the seriousness of HIV/AIDS are two major hurdles to prevention education in the black community, according to Damaris Richardson, minority outreach coordinator with the Health Education Resource Organization, Baltimore's largest AIDS education organisation.

Given the already acute shortage of health services, poor education, and the often grinding poverty that is both core and coating of life for tens of thousands of Baltimore's African-Americans, HIV is just the latest assault on an already beleaguered community. As Pridgen says, "I can't think of any area of African-American life that has not been negatively impacted [by HIV]....When you're talking about people already living on the edge, HIV will push them over."

John-Manuel Andriote, *Baltimore*

The Hardest Hit

It is, of course, dangerous to generalise about community responses to the virus. As one study summarised it: "The realities of AIDS have both provoked hostility against some groups and communities as well as broken down barriers [between others]....Personal relationships have been enriched as well as fragmented. Families, groups and communities have been strengthened as well as splintered [30]." Yet one generalisation is safer than others: the burden of caring for and supporting those affected by the disease weighs most heavily on communities already struggling with inadequate levels of health, education and employment. This is as evident in industrialised countries as it is in developing ones. In the United States, for example, two communities have been hit hardest by HIV/AIDS: relatively wealthy gay men in cities such as San Francisco and New York, and the poorer communities of African Americans and Latino Americans in cities such as Baltimore and New York. The gay community, able to draw on considerable resources of money, time and solidarity, has responded effectively to the disease on many levels, including that of reducing further transmission of the virus. The much more fragmented response in the already marginalised black community in cities like Baltimore has been very different (see Box).

"You can't do HIV education in a vacuum"

In the words of a study on community responses to HIV/AIDS: "While the 'poorest of the poor' have been notoriously hard to reach for development purposes, it has not been hard for the virus to reach them [31]." Indeed, HIV/AIDS highlights existing inequalities: in health and education services, in the situation of women, in land tenure, nutritional status, and so on. Any activities aimed at raising the standard of living of those people whose social and economic circumstances narrow their chances of protecting themselves against HIV/AIDS will help to slow the spread of the epidemic and combat its effects. Theresa Kaijage of WAMATA warns that development assistance programmes which do not tackle the inequalities in which HIV/AIDS seems to be thriving will only succeed in reinforcing the status quo [32].

CHAPTER 5

The challenge to labour

B ecause it primarily targets the most productive members of the labour force, the HIV/AIDS pandemic has profound economic implications. As the epidemic advances in developing countries, changes to the population profile will exacerbate existing skill shortages and create new ones, threatening productivity. Over time, as the young sexually active members of the labour force (20-40 years old) become infected, fewer will survive to form the older segment (40-60 years old), which has accumulated skills and experience through training and long service. This will compound the impact of the first decade of the epidemic in Africa and, to a lesser extent, in Latin America, where the higher socio-economic groups, which form the more skilled and educated section of the workforce, were disproportionately affected. Most of the research on this has been done in sub-Saharan Africa, and this chapter necessarily concentrates on this region.

In addition to the loss of labour and skills, which takes many years to replace, HIV/AIDS has implications for other aspects of employment such as training, sickness benefits, pensions and insurance. Absenteeism because of illness, caring for the sick and mourning the dead also affects productivity.

The labour force
A common image of developing countries is one of teeming cities, acting like magnets for millions of people in search of a better livelihood than the rural areas can provide. The majority of these millions remain informally employed, making a living in many different ways, working, for example, in small industries and businesses, as market traders and day labourers, brewing beer, selling food and recycling waste.

Table 1 gives some idea of the structure of the labour force in different countries. These figures, however, only really reflect the "visibly" employed: much informal employment and therefore a great deal of the work done by women would not be properly represented. This chapter focuses on formal sector employment,

Table 1: Profile of labour force in selected developing countries

	1986-89 Percentage of labour force in			1988-90 Labour force as % of total population	Women as % of labour force
	*agriculture	**industry	***services		
AFRICA					
Botswana	43.2	4.8	52.0	34.9	35.5
Nigeria	44.6	4.2	51.2	30.3	19.7
Zambia	37.9	7.8	54.9	31.5	28.7
Sudan	63.4	4.3	32.3	35.1	29.1
Kenya	81.0	6.8	12.1	40.3	40.3
Rwanda	92.8	3.0	4.3	49.2	48.0
LATIN AMERICA & THE CARIBBEAN					
Honduras	60.4	16.1	23.4	30.3	18.3
Haiti	50.4	5.7	43.9	41.1	40.0
Venezuela	12.5	17.3	70.2	35.9	21.5
Brazil	29.3	16.0	54.7	43.2	35.1
Jamaica	25.3	11.5	63.2	37.5	31.0
Guatemala	49.8	12.3	37.9	33.5	25.5
ASIA					
Singapore	0.5	29.0	70.5	48.6	39.0
Thailand	69.8	5.9	24.3	55.7	46.9
Nepal	93.0	0.6	6.5	40.5	33.8
China	73.7	13.6	12.7	59.3	43.2
India	62.6	10.8	26.6	37.9	25.6
Bangladesh	56.5	9.8	33.7	30.4	6.5

*Agriculture includes fisheries and forestry
**Industry includes manufacturing, mining, construction, energy and water works etc
***Services include trade, leisure and tourism, transport, communications, finance, medical, education, defence, welfare, domestic services etc

Source: *Human Development Report 1992*, UNDP, Table 16

not because it is the most significant but because it is more easily quantifiable and most of the research has concentrated on it: Chapter 6 covers some of the issues relevant to rural and informal employment.

Those in formal employment are the minority. The service sector dominates the picture, made up primarily of commerce centred around the export and import of goods with even the banking, finance and transport industries geared to international trade. The government is usually the next main source of employment, with hiring policies designed to absorb large numbers of unemployed school graduates. The industrial sector is typically small, based in the cities to take advantage of ports, airports and other infrastructure, financial services and government offices, and the vital but limited pool of skilled labour and management.

In spite of the accelerating drift to the cities over the last two decades, most developing countries still have a higher proportion of their population living in rural areas and working in agriculture. But HIV/AIDS, with its initial disproportionate impact on urban areas, threatens the development prospects of the commercial and industrial enterprises which are so vital to a country's economic growth. In the worst-affected countries, there is already a reduction in the supply of skilled workers, together with increased absenteeism and falling productivity. This chapter looks at the evidence and implications of this and examines the responses of some industries and organisations.

In the worst-affected countries, there is already a reduction in the supply of skilled workers

Human Resources

The impact of HIV/AIDS on the size of a country's potential labour force depends on the extent of infection and the rate at which it spreads. Anderson's model, cited in Chapter 2, takes a typical country where the potential labour force is growing at 3.6% a year. If 1% of the population is infected and the time it takes levels of HIV infection to double is 2.5 years, by year 15 of the epidemic the labour force has continued to grow but reached only 90% of what it would have been in the absence of HIV. Shortening the doubling time or increasing the seroprevalence further reduces the rate of growth. For the labour force to actually decline, however, at least 60% of the sexually active population must be infected. Current seroprevalence is far below this threshold, even in the worst-affected countries [1].

Thus, although HIV/AIDS is likely to slow the growth rate of the labour force, it is unlikely to reduce its overall size. It does, however, alter its profile, yielding a younger workforce dominated by strength and vitality but with little experience and few skills.

In many developing countries, there is already a shortage of skilled labour and a narrow and underdeveloped industrial base, exacerbated by lack of resources to overcome these problems. Many countries, particularly in parts of sub-Saharan Africa, have only one university and equally limited facilities for industrial or commercial training. Opportunities exist for further education abroad, but the high costs involved, whether borne by the state, the community or the family, severely restrict the number of people who benefit. This means that, in general, developing countries depend on the skills of a small proportion of the population; loss of these skills has tremendous implications for their economies as a whole.

Table 2: Literacy and education levels in selected developing countries

	Adult literacy as % of population aged 15+ (1990)		Average years of schooling for population aged 25+ (1990)		Number of students per 100,000 inhabitants going beyond secondary level education*
	M	F	M	F	
AFRICA					
Ghana	70	51	4.8	2.2	127
Kenya	80	59	3.2	1.3	135
Sudan	43	12	1.1	0.5	246
Zimbabwe	74	60	4.2	1.7	585
LATIN AMERICA & THE CARIBBEAN					
Brazil	83	80	4.0	1.7	585
Jamaica	98	99	5.3	5.2	556
Mexico	90	85	4.8	4.6	1,515
Venezuela	87	90	6.4	6.2	2,670
ASIA					
Bangladesh	47	22	3.1	0.9	329
Malaysia	87	70	5.6	5.0	**638
Nepal	38	13	3.2	1.0	**523
Thailand	96	90	4.3	3.3	1,734

* All figures for 1989 except those marked with ** which are 1988

Sources: Adult literacy rates and mean years of schooling taken from *Human Development Report 1992*, UNDP. Other figures from *Statistical Yearbook 1991*, UNESCO

The skill base

Most of this chapter looks at the impact of HIV/AIDS on the already skilled and educated, but there is evidence that the pool of people who will make up the next generation of skilled workers is already diminishing. Opportunities for higher education are being adversely affected. In the mid-1980s, many countries in Europe and Asia where overseas students continued their education, introduced HIV-antibody tests, deporting or refusing entry to those who tested positive. Having their course brought to an abrupt end not only caused stress and hardship for those returning home, but also meant that the money invested in their education by the state or community was lost. The number of deportations fell in the late 1980s as aspiring students underwent the test in their countries of origin. No statistics are available as to the number of potential graduates who did not apply for scholarships and grants because of their HIV-positive status, but it is likely that the numbers are not insignificant. These restrictions remain in force.

A further restraint on education may come from the number of teachers and lecturers being reduced through illness. Makerere

Table 3: The skill base—graduates in selected developing countries

	Total number of 1st degree graduates	Number of graduates per 100,000 of population	Number of graduates by selected fields of study and as % of total graduates				
			Education	Commerce	Medicine & Health	Engineering	Agriculture
AFRICA							
Ghana (1989)	1,994	14	57 3%	180 9%	127 6%	151 8%	139 7%
Kenya (1986)	2,338	11	718 31%	163 7%	157 7%	174 7%	269 12%
Zimbabwe (1986)	864	10	69 8%	164 19%	72 8%	52 6%	52 6%
LATIN AMERICA & THE CARIBBEAN							
Brazil (1988)	134,717	94	51,501 38%	34,683 26%	21,277 16%	2,158 2%	1,065 1%
Jamaica (1986)	1,823	76	133 7%	—	106 6%	132 7%	25 1%
Mexico (1989)	153,073	181	40,815 27%	26,061 17%	13,524 9%	30,087 20%	2,751 2%
ASIA							
Bangladesh (1987)	58,748	55	2,709 5%	8,882 15%	1,055 2%	742 1%	673 1%
Nepal (1988)	26,847	149	2,870 11%	8,925 33%	256 1%	376 1%	724 3%
Thailand (1988)	66,954	124	22,608 34%	10,158 15%	4,871 7%	2,617 4%	3,883 6%

Sources: Information from *Statistical Yearbook 1991*, UNESCO; population figures from *Human Development Report 1990*, UNDP, and *World Development Report 1988, 1989 and 1991*, World Bank

"The most University in Uganda reports that so far 25 of its students have
expert died of AIDS, and at Kyambogo teachers' training college there
go first" have been 22 deaths from AIDS [2].
Tables 2 and 3 indicate the education and skill base in a number
of countries in the developing world. Table 2 compares male and
female literacy and schooling levels. In almost every country
women are less literate and complete fewer years of schooling
than men. These inequalities are reflected in employment
patterns: Table 1 shows women as a percentage of the workforce.
Men are more likely to be in formal employment, to have security
in employment and to receive training.
Table 3 shows the numbers and the proportion of the
population graduating in different disciplines in selected
countries. Africa has a very narrow skill base, with few
disciplines producing more than 100 graduates each year in most
countries. Prisca Tembo, of Botswana's "AIDS in the workplace"
campaign, emphasises the potential difficulties for countries with
a shortage of skilled workers: "Even without AIDS, Botswana
does not have enough local engineers, architects, accountants and
business managers [3]." Because in Asia a higher proportion of
the population take degrees, the skill base is broader. It is higher
still in Latin America and the Caribbean, suggesting that the
impact on this sector will be less severe.

Impact on Skilled Labour

In the first decade of the epidemic in sub-Saharan Africa there
has been a disproportionate incidence of infection in those with
higher education, income and skill levels. A 1988 study in Zaire
found higher HIV infection rates in better educated and higher
paid male workers: 5% compared with 3% in workers in lower
positions, a finding backed up by other research in the country
[4]. A national survey in Rwanda found an infection rate of almost
30% in urban adults with secondary schooling, compared to
20.8% among those with less schooling [5]. A 1985 study in
Zambia found 8% infection among those with fewer than five
years of schooling, rising to 33.3% of those with 14 or more years
[6]. Another study in Rwanda—on urban women—found a
similar correlation but one which highlights the inequalities of
gender. Researchers found there was a significant correlation
between the women's HIV status and their partners' education
and income, much stronger than any correlation with the
women's own socio-economic status. Eighteen per cent of
women whose partners had less than five years of schooling were

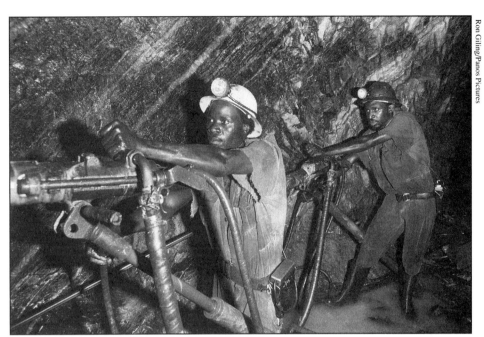

Zambia's copper mining industry produces 75% of the country's export earnings and depends on a small group of skilled workers. Illness and death in this workforce have severe implications for the national economy.

HIV positive, compared to 34% of women with partners who had eight or more years of education. Moreover, seroprevalence among women whose partners had no monthly income was 22%, compared to 25% for those whose partners earned up to $100 a month and 35% for those whose partners earned $100 or more a month [7].

The Zaire study examines the background to such statistics: "Having a higher income means having to be less reliant on a transportation system which can entail a 2-3 hour journey each way to work. This difference in disposable income and leisure time and the increased opportunity for sexual activity which it could provide may partially explain the higher HIV-1 seroprevalence...in higher-paid employees [8]."

This same pattern is repeated in other countries. Describing the impact of sickness and death caused by the epidemic, Peter Fraser-Mackenzie of Zimbabwe's Commercial Farmers Union (CFU) suggests that "the most expert go first [9]". A Zambian survey of a number of parastatal organisations found that "AIDS tended to hit their support staff and middle management workers the hardest [10]".

A report on the Zambian copper-mining industry, which earns 75% of the country's foreign exchange, stated that "the danger is that skilled workers, supervisors and managers will die of AIDS faster than replacements can be trained. The result will not be a

The sugar industry in Swaziland

Swaziland is a small (17,364 sq km) landlocked country in Southern Africa. It has a population of only 800,000, 80% of which lives in the rural areas. In 1990/91, agriculture accounted for 17.5% of the gross domestic product (GDP), more than half of which was provided by large sugar estates. In addition, sugar milling accounts for 26% of manufacturing output, and links with the rest of the economy increase its importance further. In 1988, some 89,000 Swazi were in formal sector employment. Of these 23,500 were in agriculture, of whom about 10,000 worked on sugar estates and in the mills.

The large estates operate as fairly closed communities, providing housing, medical services and a number of other benefits. Company housing is of relatively high quality, with water and electricity provided. Permanent workers occupy housing until they retire or are discharged, when they must leave the estate. Seasonal and casual workers are also employed.

Swaziland reported its first case of AIDS in 1987. The first national survey, in 1990, found that 2.4% of women attending antenatal clinics were HIV-positive. Sugar company medical services surveying antenatal clinics in the first three months of 1992 found a consistent rate of 9% seropositivity. Medical officers and senior management on the estates are extremely concerned about the HIV epidemic. Although the number of cases has been small so far, they are a worrying indication of potential difficulties, both in terms of company benefits and productivity.

Company benefits include health care, housing, and training. In theory, when employees fall ill and can no longer work, they are given a medical discharge and have to leave the estate. All terminal benefits are paid out and company responsibility ends. In these circumstances, HIV would not be a significant drain on company resources. But as one senior officer noted: "Can we afford to do this? What will the effect be on the company image if the Swazi see it working people until they can no longer function and then throwing them off the estate? Equally, we cannot afford to have scarce housing tied up."

One option currently being examined is to make a contract with the Swaziland Hospice movement to care for dying patients at their homes off the estates. This would cost approximately $600 per case and would be a realistic and compassionate response. The real drain on benefits will come from the dependants, who are entitled to free health care and—if they die while their spouse or parent is in company employ—to a free coffin and transport for the burial.

It is generally felt that the costs of the epidemic may be bearable for the next few years, but as more of those already infected fall ill, the pressure on staff, budgets and facilities will become insupportable. Training departments will also have to consider the impact of HIV/AIDS. Far-sighted companies will increase the number of trainees to ensure that they are not left short of crucial skilled manpower. This will mean increasing budgets.

A consultancy report prepared for one of the main companies, in March/April 1992, concluded that AIDS would not have an immediate effect on productivity, partly because it will be several years before significant numbers begin to fall ill and die. So far, of 3,100 employees, only five have died and two are ill.

Even when HIV/AIDS starts to make deep inroads into the pool of employees, there is enough surplus labour available to ensure that workers at the lower end of the skill spectrum are replaced. The real problem arises from the loss of skilled and professional staff. These may be difficult to replace from within Swaziland, which may mean expensive

expatriates have to be employed, reversing the gains made by the use of local staff. The challenge to the sugar companies is to respond to HIV/AIDS in a compassionate but cost-effective way—a way which will balance the obligations to employees, society and the shareholders, and ensure that one of the main components of the Swazi economy is able to continue functioning, and contribute to national development.
Alan Whiteside, *University of Natal, South Africa*, and **Ian Gilbertson**, *senior medical officer at a sugar estate, Swaziland*

sudden collapse in mine output. Rather there will be a slow but steady increase in the incidence of breakdowns, accidents, delays and misjudgements and output will suffer [11]."

Although few studies on the relationship between skill levels and HIV prevalence in other regions have been undertaken, the evidence suggests that in Latin America, in the early stages, the epidemic primarily targeted richer, better educated gay men; now it is increasingly poorer, unskilled men (and women) who are most affected [12]. In Asia, anecdotal evidence suggests HIV/AIDS predominantly affects the poor and unskilled.

Loss of Productivity

HIV/AIDS causes loss of productivity in many ways. As a disease characterised by periods of illness, it leads to absenteeism when people are sick and caring for the sick. According to Fraser-Mackenzie, "sickness [from HIV/AIDS] is a greater cost [to a company] than deaths," and he adds that the early picture of the epidemic has revealed increased "absenteeism, tiredness and intermittent sickness [13]". "The biggest problem is the loss of production hours due to the off days given to [sickness resulting from AIDS]," reported one Zambian manager [14]. The human resources director of Medscheme, Gary Taylor, found that a number of South African employers in his study on the medical schemes movement had reached the conclusion that: "The financial and logistical costs of AIDS illness at work will be more onerous than actual death in service [15]."

Such anecdotal evidence is widespread, but has not yet been matched by published research into the relationship between an individual's HIV status and their productivity. It is an area which needs further study, although there are difficulties in trying to measure the effects of bouts of illness on lost output, as attempts to do the same for malaria—a classic example of a debilitating disease which impairs productivity—have found [16].

In some countries in Africa productivity is being affected by increased funeral attendance, a social obligation which provides

"Sickness from HIV/AIDS is a greater cost to a company than deaths"

The cost to companies in Uganda

Eleven years after HIV/AIDS appeared in Uganda, the disease is devastating workplaces and there are reports that in some parastatal organisations hundreds of employees have already died. No parastatal has felt the effects of HIV/AIDS more fully than the Uganda Railway Corporation (URC). According to the Danish International Development Agency (DANIDA), which made a comprehensive report on URC last year, 10% of URC's 5,600 employees may have died of AIDS in the past few years. HIV/AIDS has become one of the causes of high labour turnover, now running at 15% per year.

To some URC executives, the figure of 10% seems exaggerated. Ephrance Kabatangale, the corporation's principal public relations officer, comments: "I don't deny that AIDS is a serious problem but the 10% is just too much." But URC's principal medical officer seems to concur with the information. "I haven't seen the report but I agree entirely with these figures and it could even be higher. It is spreading faster because of the nature of our industry," he explained. "We are in the transport business, where some of our workers take three weeks away from home." He paused. "You know that old habits die hard and some people can't stay all that long without a woman." He added that recently many of the railway workers, on average three a month, have wanted early retirement. "We have been testing them for a number of diseases including, of course, AIDS....all of them have been testing HIV-positive." The corporation then advises them to opt for lighter jobs. But since many of them insist on leaving, they are allowed to retire with all benefits.

In the Uganda Posts and Telecommunications Corporation (UPTC) workers say that at least 50 employees, including two senior staff members, died last year. But Francis Kanyeihamba, UPTC's public relations officer, says it is difficult to determine whether all these employees died of AIDS. Besides direct loss of employees, some government offices are recording high rates of absenteeism. Edward Wasswa, an employee in the Ministry of Commerce and Industry, says: "Even if someone does not die here, every week we have at least three employees asking for permission to attend a relative's funeral." In some departments, if the death is of someone senior, whole offices will be empty.

The results have been devastating to many agencies and companies that are struggling to make a profit after years of disruption and inefficiency. But the most notable problem has been the increase in medical costs. DANIDA reported that the URC has been faced with high hospital bills. "The hospital bill now takes 77.3 million shillings [$77,300] every year from URC coffers. It has definitely raised the amount of money spent on individuals. On average URC now spends 303,924 shillings ($300) on an individual; in 1988 the corporation spent an average of 69,621 shillings ($69). For a corporation with revenue of $6.1 million a year, this could affect its financial status."

Some workplaces have been forced into cruel decisions. British American Tobacco (BAT), for example, now subjects its workers or would-be employees to blood tests. But this has triggered criticism among the employees. One said, "This is a violation of what WHO says—that there should be no discrimination against AIDS victims."

Many government officials say that if nothing is done the country will face an acute manpower problem in virtually all sectors; some say that Uganda could lose up to 300 civil servants by 1995 at current rates of infection. This would be disastrous in government departments which already have many unfilled vacancies.

Crespo Sebunya, *Kampala*

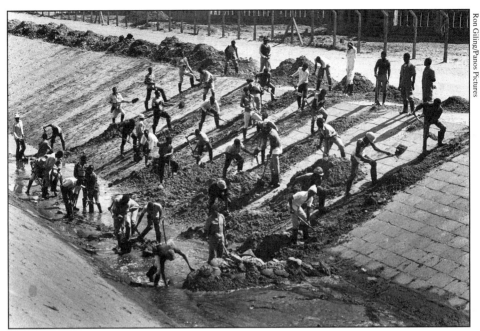

important support to families and communities but which may involve several days off work. The manager of one Ugandan company wrote to his head office, "There are days lost for funerals of non-staff members, there are days lost and costs of funerals when staff members or their immediate family die. What policy do we have to contribute to these costs? Should we be increasing our compassionate leave allowance of five days per year? Should we be putting a 'cost' element in our budget [17]?"

Caring for those who are ill is a further source of absenteeism. "As AIDS strikes mothers and household heads, secondary workers [not the primary breadwinner] will have to withdraw from the labor force to take care of the ill as hospitalization will be available for only a small number. Secondary workers also will have to bear the burden of caring for the children and elderly dependants of AIDS victims," was the conclusion of one report on sub-Saharan Africa [18].

Not surprisingly, the wide range of psychological reactions to HIV/AIDS in the workplace also creates problems. The company manager quoted above went on to write: "These...problems are not only those of the individual and his/her relationship to his/her colleagues, but the relationship of groups (who assume themselves to be negative) to individuals or groups whom they know or believe to be positive. For instance the manager of [a major company] in Kampala recently told me he had been

Large-scale construction projects employ huge numbers of men, often away from their homes. Companies which provide STD awareness campaigns as well as condoms can do much to reduce the spread of HIV/AIDS.

"Finding and retraining workers to replace those who have died will be difficult and costly"

asked/forced by his local staff to sack three tea boys/girls known to be HIV-positive....even though we assume some of the members of the pressure group are positive themselves [19]."

Implications

Almost every aspect of formal sector employment must be re-examined in the light of HIV/AIDS, including training, sickness and unemployment benefits, insurance and pensions.

More extensive training will be needed to take account of possible future shortfalls in skill levels. Ellis Smith, chairman of the Federation of Master Printers in Zimbabwe, has said that greater numbers of apprentices should be recruited by the printing industry to replace those who will die of AIDS [20]. The Thai study cited in Chapter 2 suggests that "finding and retraining workers to replace those who have died will be difficult and costly, especially if the unemployment rate remains at the current low 3%-4% level [21]".

Fraser-Mackenzie of Zimbabwe's CFU suggests that the financial cost of ill health and the benefits given at the termination of employment will have to be reviewed. The formal labour force may become younger and include more women. One change that has already been observed in Zimbabwe is the increasing cultivation of chillies because they can be harvested easily by children [22].

Major construction projects such as dams and roads, which bring large numbers of men to often isolated rural sites, which then attract prostitutes, may also contribute to the spread of HIV/AIDS. It has been suggested that the companies and donor agencies involved should build in the cost of condom provision and awareness programmes. Where this has been done, there has been a striking decrease in STDs among staff [23].

Responses

There is growing international recognition that all levels of formal sector employment must respond to the threat of HIV/AIDS, although there may not be consensus on the nature of that response. Commerce, industry, government and the service sector contain many different kinds of institutions, managed by individuals whose decisionmaking will be influenced by different criteria. Broadly speaking, reactions to the epidemic form a spectrum which at one end seeks to exclude all HIV/AIDS-related costs and at the other recognises that such costs are inevitable. The three areas in which the impact of HIV/AIDS is likely to be most acute are recruitment, training and employment benefits.

Pensions and insurance in Southern Africa

The extent of health and life insurance and pension schemes in any country is restricted by the formal sector base on which it stands. Whether provided by the state or private companies, pensions and insurance are a form of capital through which individuals can secure incomes for themselves or their families in the event of death, disability or old age. Provision of both pensions and insurance comes from contributions by those in work; calculating the benefits available is a complex process which is extremely sensitive to variations in contributions and demands for benefits by those entitled.

Insurance companies face enormous losses unless they can limit their liability. Before HIV/AIDS, they anticipated that a typical 30-year-old taking out life insurance would pay premiums for 30-40 years; now they might pay for only five years before dying of AIDS. Faced by increasing numbers of claims as a result of illness or death from AIDS, many insurance companies in the North have amended policies to exclude payment for illness or death caused by the disease or have refused to insure individuals they believe to be at risk. In many countries there has been considerable opposition to such action, from those who believe it discriminates unnecessarily and from health authorities which believe that it is likely to increase spread of the virus by deterring people from being tested.

In the South, where a smaller proportion of the population is covered by insurance, the question of the impact of the epidemic has been most widely studied in Southern Africa. In 1985-88, South African life insurance companies paid a total of Rand 3.3 million ($1.3 million) in AIDS-related claims. In 1989 alone, payments were R2.7 million ($1.06 million). The insurance industry in South Africa requires applicants for policies over R200,000 ($79,000 in 1989) to have an HIV test or sign a waiver exempting the company from payment in AIDS-related cases [41]. Many South African companies have reduced the policy limit to half this, in some cases to R50,000 [42], and it is recommended that they regularly review the limit. A similar policy is adopted in Zimbabwe, and in several African countries where testing is not permitted, life cover is no longer available [43].

In Zimbabwe, although government policy prevented doctors from identifying AIDS as a cause of death until December 1989, claims in group life schemes of a major insurance company doubled between 1986 and 1990, while the amount paid out multiplied 25-fold [44]. In December 1989, Zimbabwean insurance companies reached an agreement with the government which allowed them to require an HIV test from anyone seeking a life policy over Z$100,000 ($44,000 in 1989), a relatively high amount. If someone who tests negative subsequently dies of AIDS, the company has to pay the beneficiary. In Malawi, Old Mutual tested all applicants until the government prohibited insurance companies from doing so; the company has since withdrawn from the Malawi market.

Recruitment

Companies which follow a strict policy of excluding HIV/AIDS from the workplace screen all potential employees, refuse to hire those who are HIV-positive, and dismiss employees discovered to be carrying the virus. An example of the "exclusion" approach comes from the South African Chamber of Mines which in the late 1980s introduced pre-employment testing and refused to recruit those who tested HIV-positive. According to a senior

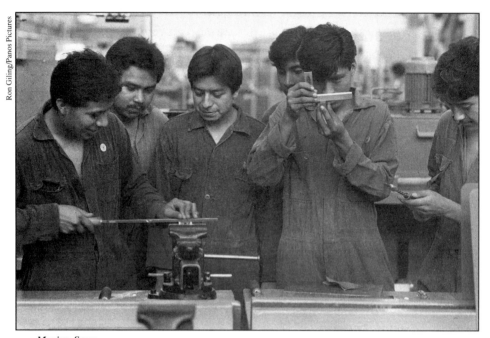

Ron Giling/Panos Pictures

Mexico. Some companies are reluctant to train workers without screening out those with HIV, yet most people testing positive would have many years of productive life ahead of them.

general manager: "AIDS is costly for the mining industry and for the families involved since very often it is the able-bodied and breadwinners who are infected. If we lose miners, technicians or any other staff through AIDS, then we have to train new people to do the job and this is costly [24]." The Malawian government's response to this approach was to prohibit its nationals from working in the South African mines.

The Zambian survey of 10 parastatal companies indicated that six required prospective employees to be tested for HIV and refused employment to those discovered to be positive. Four companies would not send employees with HIV/AIDS for training, but none would dismiss an employee discovered to be infected [25]. Despite the government policy against any form of pre- or post-employment HIV testing, many companies in Zimbabwe screen potential recruits: a 1991 survey of 94 companies revealed that 21 already carry out such screening, while a further 28 thought that some form of screening was a good idea [26].

The legality of pre-employment screening varies from country to country, but in practical terms it is viable only in countries with a broad skill base and low rates of infection, where there is a strong likelihood of finding HIV-negative recruits with the relevant skills. In countries with a narrow skill base and high rates of infection, exclusion is likely to be a self-defeating policy —particularly since the long incubation period of the disease means that the majority of those infected will have many years of productive work ahead of them. Helen Jackson of the AIDS Counselling Trust, a Zimbabwean NGO, points out: "If screening is used to block infected people from employment, thousands of fit men and women will be unemployed and unemployable, and their skills, training and experience wasted [27]."

"To test or not to test? That is the basic question"

In addition, the nature of HIV/AIDS means that those who contract it in the six months prior to pre-employment testing may give a negative result.

Training and staff development
In a number of countries there is debate on whether to test employees prior to training and, by analogy, to test students offered further education scholarships. It has been suggested that such testing may be justified since money is to be invested in a person which will only be paid back over time; if the employee falls sick soon after completing the training, the investment will have been lost. A counter argument from Zimbabwe's Minister of Health is that employees remain with a company for an average of only three years after they are trained [28]; since people with HIV can remain healthy for much longer periods, there appears no justification for discriminating against them. Helen Jackson points out: "Screening...does not indicate when a person contracted the HIV virus. With most training programmes, the employer could still get a return, because people may still have a fairly long work life ahead of them [29]."

Alan Whiteside of the University of Natal, South Africa, and author of several reports on the economic implications of HIV/AIDS in Southern Africa, has noted that "some companies and governments are insisting that trainees going on lengthy overseas courses be tested and there is compelling logic for this if the course exceeds three or four years [30]." To justify this, however, a cost-benefit analysis would have to compare the costs of the training with the likely return from the individual; such an analysis would also have to take into account the probability of death and disability occurring from other diseases or circumstances.

Employment benefits
Pre-employment testing may miss a recent infection or an employee may become become infected after being hired. The reaction and responsibility of companies towards HIV-positive employees varies. Where HIV infection has been or is a relatively

The multinational response

"If you are not prepared to employ HIV-positive people in Africa, you might as well shut up shop and go away."

"We normally have 2%-3% labour turnover. But if 25% of the labour force is HIV-positive, we may have a major staffing problem in the future."

"In the end we are a commercial organisation, and may have to balance the humane and the pragmatic."

"To test or not to test? That is the basic question."

"You cannot expect the taxpayers of Europe and America to pay for health care in Africa."

These statements were all made by senior officials of various multinational companies operating in Africa, except for the last, which was made by Edward Jaycox, vice-president for Africa of the World Bank [45]. The comments indicate the range of issues raised by HIV/AIDS for multinationals in Africa.

Three large multinationals—BAT, Unilever and BP Africa—have thought hard about the policies they should adopt. Two of the three have established a set of guidelines about how local managers should react to the disease. There are clear directives stating that there is no justification for HIV screening and there should be no discrimination against HIV-positive people in employment or hiring. The third company is actively debating its guideline document. All three companies stress that local managers in each country are required to operate within the law of that country, where specific legislation against screening or discrimination exists.

It seems that these multinationals, and possibly others, may be following a more ethical line than many local private or parastatal companies in East and Central Africa, some of which admit to screening potential employees for HIV. It may also be the case that guidelines have been drawn up in part with an eye to public reaction and attitudes in the country where their headquarters is based, rather than to reflect local conditions. Such guidelines are often meant to apply globally, which may mean they are not totally suitable for Africa.

Other factors also operate. Where a person is being recruited by a multinational to a managerial job which may require him/her to travel to countries which have strict rules about testing incomers for HIV, that applicant may be screened. And company officials admitted informally that if HIV/AIDS and its associated medical costs were to have an impact on "the bottom line"—profitability—different policies may be adopted.

Furthermore, actions may differ from policy. Local managers often have wide discretion over the application of company policy. They may decide to screen some or all job applicants for HIV without telling head office. A local company doctor, who may not be a company employee, may test a job applicant for HIV without telling the local manager and use a positive result as a reason for recommending that they be turned down.

There is growing pressure from local managers in Africa to have clear corporate guidelines laid down for them by headquarters on such matters as:

• Can they recruit extra workers to make up for the expected loss of employees to AIDS?

• Should they invest in extra machinery to make up for the skilled workforce lost to AIDS?

• What public relations policy should they adopt in a case where, for example, a food processing plant is reported to have an HIV-positive employee? What do you tell the media and the public?

Unilever has 80,000 employees in Africa, of whom about 2,000 are managers. Of these some 150 are expatriates, including 30 who come from other parts of the continent. The company has what it describes as "guidelines rather than a formal policy" and takes an active monitoring and educational role in relation to AIDS. Chairmen of local companies have been asked, in formulating their five-year business plans, to consider whether HIV/AIDS would affect their markets—either their size or the consumer patterns.

BP Africa has a formal "common agreed policy" on AIDS, written into its employee relations handbook. The company points out that, being in the oil business, many of its staff are pump attendants or drivers or mix with delivery drivers—and are therefore seen as high-risk groups. In response, BP has conducted large-scale educational campaigns among its staff. In Zimbabwe this includes giving every employee a booklet entitled *AIDS: let's fight it together*, available in English and vernacular languages. This will be supplemented by a video on AIDS prevention made locally, specifically for industry.

The company points out that sometimes the only suitable candidate for a job may be HIV-positive, so both ethics and practicality favour the employment of that person for as long as they are fit to work.

Rex Winsbury, *editor, AIDS Analysis Africa*

recent phenomenon, there are frequent reports of employees being dismissed on suspicion or evidence of infection [31]. Where the epidemic is already widespread and recognised, company response tends to be more sympathetic.

The approach emerging in companies that have debated and adopted HIV/AIDS policies is to treat the disease like any other life-threatening illness. Employees thus continue to work as long as they are able to do so, at which point they are retired on grounds of ill health. In the meantime, they receive the same benefits as any other employees. However, the extent of employment benefits may alter as a result of HIV/AIDS. Where seroprevalence rates are high, companies may consider setting financial limits to employment benefits; such limits may be acceptable if they are negotiated with employees, consistent and known in advance. Tony Devlin of Anglo-American Zimbabwe makes two suggestions: setting up accurate attendance registers and reviewing medical, pension and disability benefits. The completion of attendance registers is necessary in order to pick up absences due to HIV infection [32].

Policy Issues
Government support is essential to encourage formulation of HIV/AIDS policies; in both Thailand and Zimbabwe prominent government officials have been outspoken on the issue of HIV/AIDS. The International Labour Organization has also recommended that "consistent [HIV/AIDS] policies and

procedures should be developed at national and enterprise levels through consultations between workers, employers and their organizations, and where appropriate, governmental agencies and other organizations [33]."

Organised labour (trade unions) is also beginning to respond to the epidemic. The policy of the Zimbabwe Congress of Trade Unions (ZCTU) is that HIV-positive people should be protected from all forms of isolation or victimisation, and that their status should be confidential. Workers should not be tested for employment, training or promotion purposes. There should be no HIV testing or discrimination with regard to pensions, health and medical insurance, access to housing loans, and insurance. Clauses should be included in collective bargaining agreements to prevent HIV testing at the workplace and keep HIV status confidential. Legislation should be passed to ensure these policies on HIV/AIDS and employment are adhered to [34]. It is unclear what priority ZCTU will give HIV/AIDS. As Whiteside points out, its response is likely to be overshadowed by other problems such as unemployment and wage protection. Although the ZCTU has a substantial membership in Zimbabwe's formal workforce, the preponderance of men may mean that women's rights will not be addressed as urgently as needed [35].

A situation where some companies maintain an "exclusion" policy and others do not test is likely to lead to the latter companies being burdened with comparatively higher costs. The solution may be for legislation to ensure that all commercial enterprises adopt the same policy.

Ben Chirwa of the Health Education Unit of the Zambian Ministry of Health has said that while the initial response of some companies to HIV/AIDS was "panic", the same companies have now worked out consistent policies and education programmes [36]. For example, even in countries with a broad skill base, where "exclusion" policies are theoretically more viable, company policies and state legislation have tended towards the opposite approach. Anti-discrimination policies already exist or are being drawn up in a number of countries. In the United States, for example, city or state measures protecting the rights of people with HIV have been supplemented by the 1990 Americans with Disabilities Act, which covers a wide range of situations in which HIV/AIDS might be an issue, without specifically referring to the disease [37].

Industry as Educators

"Dead customers don't buy"

It makes economic sense for industry and commerce to adopt HIV/AIDS policies, and to encompass not only the reactive steps just described, but also proactive measures such as education programmes designed to limit the spread of HIV among the workforce. The expense of such programmes is minimal compared with the costs of replacing someone who dies of the illness (see Chapter 8).

The Confederation of Zimbabwe Industries, for example, has established an AIDS committee and is trying to get its members actively involved in raising AIDS awareness. Companies are trying to place counsellors in the workforce and to encourage the use of condoms. According to Alan Whiteside: "Collective business has to put pressure on government for an intensive AIDS education campaign and in addition set up their own regional education centres where employees live [38]." Some examples of company education programmes are described in this chapter and in Chapter 8.

Organised labour also has a role to play in education on HIV/AIDS issues. The Argentinian General Labour Federation (CGT) is developing a programme of training union representatives as HIV/AIDS educators, aiming to have 400 in place in 1992 and 10 times that number in 1993. The fact that educators are fellow-workers rather than management staff makes them more likely to be listened to and trusted. It is also seen as a way of encouraging solidarity and communication on a subject which can so easily lead to marginalisation, and empowering workers by giving them responsibility for an issue which affects everyone. In the words of metalworker Luis Hernandez: "When I hear people talk about AIDS I used to think that it was important to talk to doctors about how to avoid it. Now I can't get used to the fact that it is me that my workmates consult. Me, who only passed fourth grade [39]!"

Wider implications

The current picture, with some regional variation, is that HIV/AIDS threatens to create particularly damaging shortages in skilled labour but will increasingly affect the unskilled, the less educated and those employed in the informal sector and in the rural areas.

Many developing countries are already struggling with worsening economic conditions. If the effect of the epidemic is to erode further their hopes of industrial or commercial development, it is likely that even greater numbers of people will

Thai industry: "enlightened self-interest"

"In AIDS prevention, a businessman is more useful than a hospital," says Chookiat Prateeptong, human resources manager for Robinson's Department Stores in Thailand. "A businessman can prevent, say, 100 deaths, which a hospital cannot do."

To know that 70% of Robinson's 3,700 employees are under 21 years old and 60% are women is to understand the company's concern. In cooperation with a local non-government organisation (NGO), Robinson's has educated all its employees about AIDS. It also provides lectures on other health topics. As Chookiat Prateeptong explains, AIDS prevention is only one part of the company's broad corporate objectives of ensuring their employees' welfare.

With about 600,000 people currently HIV-positive in Thailand and an estimated increase of 1,000 new infections a day, few companies will escape unscathed over the next decade. Transmission is predominantly heterosexual and the widespread use of commercial sex by most Thai men makes HIV an "equal opportunity" infection, both in the boardroom and on the factory floor.

The extent of the epidemic raises concern among company managers about high outlays on medical benefits. Although not required to provide such benefits for their employees, most large companies do so and their contribution could be critical in alleviating the burden of HIV/AIDS on the government. However, such contributions might become limited. As the managing director of one multinational corporation says, "We are happy to help with the first three or four cases, but frankly if it becomes more than that, I'm not sure what we can afford to do." Well-known companies have dismissed employees on learning about their HIV status, although the stated reasons have usually been different. Many companies fear the loss of trained and experienced employees, especially as they are harder to find after a decade of booming economic growth in Thailand. The manager of a hotel chain put it in perspective: "I'm not so worried about losing my training investment to AIDS; I'm more afraid of losing staff to the competition after I have spent $2,000 per head to train them."

In spite of the potential increase in medical costs and other losses, only a few companies have initiated AIDS prevention programmes. Many managers who wish to take action are unsure about what steps they should take: a multinational advertising agency which helped the government and a local NGO launch a mass media AIDS education campaign, has yet to begin its own formal in-house education.

Several NGOs provide such a service, but cannot meet all the requests for their help. In addition, even when workers have been given AIDS information, often through lectures and slide shows, the managers have not been informed about how to manage AIDS in the workplace or how to continue the education activities. The situation is improving with the emergence of a new NGO, the AIDS Trust of Thailand, which is establishing a professional service to meet the demand. "AIDS education must be tailored to match each employee audience," says Puangpayom Yuvaboon, training manager for the Dusit Thani Hotel in Bangkok. "We found that by combining the knowledge and skills of private business, government offices and community-based groups, we can deliver AIDS education programmes that appeal to all our staff, regardless of their past education or previous training experience."

Some companies started AIDS prevention activities after finding they had HIV-positive members of staff. Taken by surprise, they adopted a crisis response, often including unnecessary and even damaging measures. However, such panic measures seem to be decreasing and many companies who at one time tested or dismissed staff have adopted a more reasonable approach. One automobile assembly company with 5,000 employees, who had found one employee HIV-positive, discontinued mandatory blood testing after employee protest. Meanwhile government guidelines emphasise that testing must be voluntary and confidential, HIV-positive employees should be retained and supported, and companies should try to educate their staff and customers.

Many companies' motivation does spring from genuine concern about the situation, although others operate from "enlightened self-interest". As Mechai Viravaidya, chairman of the NGO Population and Community Development Association and a minister in the Prime Minister's office, says: "Dead customers don't buy!"

Corporations form an important part of Thailand's AIDS prevention efforts. Business representatives are active members of the National AIDS Committee and corporate logos appear on AIDS information posters and leaflets, as well as in television and radio spots on AIDS. American International Insurance printed information leaflets for its millions of policyholders and for general distribution by NGOs. A beverage company, Krating Daeng, printed AIDS information for distribution with its popular soft drink. Kodak provided slide shows for factories, schools and villages. Saatchi and Saatchi Advertising has produced television and radio spots for the Prime Minister's office, which coordinates AIDS prevention activities at the national level.

Some companies contribute to larger-scale efforts in exchange for assistance with their own in-house needs. The Thai Farmers Bank supported a $200,000 package for an NGO to hire HIV-positive AIDS educators, to talk to the bank's staff and representatives from its top 200 corporate clients, to study the impact of AIDS on the Thai economy, to provide economic opportunities to women in poor villages in Northern Thailand who might otherwise be forced into prostitution, and to establish a counselling centre for HIV-positive people.

Population and Community Development Association, *Bangkok*

be pushed towards more informal economic activities. There will be increased movement of labour not only between the formal and informal sectors but also between rural and urban areas. Migration may become not only a contributing factor to the spread of the epidemic but also a consequence, as deaths within a family, loss of land or unemployment force survivors to seek a livelihood elsewhere.

Declines in formal sector employment and in the value of wages have already increased dependence on income from the informal sector. In Africa, urban unemployment rates in the formal sector rose from about 10% in the mid-1970s to about 30% in the mid-1980s, while informal sector employment increased by 6.7%. Women increasingly form the majority of those in the informal sector: rising from 56% in 1985 to 66% in 1990 in many African countries [40].

This chapter has concentrated on the effect of HIV/AIDS on

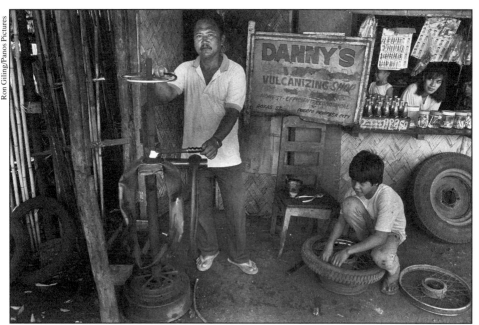

Ron Giling/Panos Pictures

In many developing countries, the informal economy is where most people work. Small businesses like this one in the Phillipines do not make much impact on national statistics, but widespread loss of labour and income from HIV/AIDS at this level will affect the livelihoods of millions.

skilled labour and formal sector employment but as the above makes clear, most developing countries have a large and growing informal sector, which is more difficult to measure in economic terms but is nevertheless extremely significant in terms of their population's employment and income. Although the prevalence rate of HIV/AIDS is currently higher in towns and cities and, in sub-Saharan Africa, among skilled as opposed to unskilled male workers, it has the potential to become a disease of the rural poor. Since this group forms the majority of the population in developing countries, the overall numbers of those affected by HIV/AIDS will rise. And since most people in the rural areas are involved in food production, the implications are considerable. The next chapter looks at the potential effect on the rural labour force and on food security.

CHAPTER 6

Rural households and food security

The greatest resource for the majority of small farmers throughout the world is their own labour. HIV/AIDS directly attacks that resource, eroding the physical energy of those with the disease and absorbing the time and energy of those who care for them. With many small farmers surviving on a knife edge, loss of labour from HIV/AIDS can tip the balance and send them into a downward spiral of diminishing food production and income, and ever increasing poverty.

While HIV remains more prevalent in urban areas, a rise in rural infection rates has been seen in a number of countries in recent years; unofficial reports suggest 20% in some areas. An average rate of 10% would imply the loss of one or two adults per household, which has already happened in parts of Uganda. One study in East Africa predicts that this rate of infection could result in the loss of 25% of the rural labour force [1].

The pattern of HIV infection in rural areas generally reflects opportunities for transmission of the virus: high near trading centres and on transport routes, and low in communities where there is little movement of population [2]. The practice of seasonal or semi-permanent migration to industrial or urban centres also facilitates the spread of HIV to rural communities. Even if rural infection rates remain lower than in urban areas, the fact that the majority of the population in the developing world lives outside the cities (see Table 1) means that the overall number of those affected is likely to be higher. And since most of them would be engaged in agriculture, the loss of their labour has major implications for food and cash crop production. HIV/AIDS is already having an effect: in parts of Kagera, Tanzania, where some 30,000 people have died because of AIDS and more than 70% of those were men and women aged between 20 and 40 years, agricultural production is reported to have fallen from previous levels by 3% to 20% [3].

Table 1: Percentage of population in rural areas

	1960	1990	2000
AFRICA			
Swaziland	96	67	55
Cameroon	86	59	49
Senegal	68	62	55
Mozambique	96	73	59
Ethiopia	94	87	83
Zimbabwe	87	72	65
Tanzania	95	67	53
The Gambia	87	77	70
LATIN AMERICA			
& THE CARIBBEAN			
Guatemala	68	61	56
Uruguay	20	14	13
Colombia	52	30	25
Bolivia	61	49	42
Honduras	77	56	48
Dominican Republic	70	40	32
Jamaica	66	48	41
Mexico	49	27	23
ASIA			
Bangladesh	95	84	77
Nepal	97	90	86
India	82	73	68
Myanmar	81	75	72
Pakistan	78	68	62
Indonesia	85	69	60
Thailand	87	77	71
Korea, Rep. of	72	28	19

Source: *Human Development Report 1992*, UNDP, Table 21

A Vital Industry

Agriculture is a vital component of the economies of most developing countries, providing national income, export earnings, employment, food and raw materials for industry. In sub-Saharan Africa, agriculture accounted for 32% of the region's gross domestic product (GDP) and 29% of its export revenues in 1990. In some of these countries agricultural produce provided over 90% of export earnings. In South Asia, agriculture provided 33% of GDP and 24% of export earnings. These figures compare with 10% and 29% respectively for Latin America and the Caribbean in the same year (1990) [4].

Staple food crops are generally grown for domestic consumption while cash crops are grown for export. Usually the latter are non-food crops such as tobacco, cotton or palm oil, or food crops which need further processing such as cacao, coffee and tea. A high percentage of export crops is grown on plantations and large commercial farms, but the proportion varies. In Uganda, the main export crop—coffee—is predominantly grown on small farms, while in Malawi large farms dominate production of the main export crops: tobacco, tea and sugar. Overall, however, the bulk of agricultural production in Africa is heavily labour-intensive and takes place on small family farms. Because these farms will be badly affected by the loss of working adults and because of the high rates of HIV/AIDS in many of the countries of East and Central Africa, several studies have been undertaken to assess the possible impact on farm labour and production in the region.

A rise in rural infection rates has been seen in a number of countries

Tipping the balance?

Even before the advent of HIV/AIDS, food security in Africa was under threat. Drought, environmental mismanagement, social and political unrest, export-oriented agricultural policies and population growth are some of the factors which have meant that food production has been declining over the last 20 years. Per capita consumption in 1980 was almost 20% below what it was at the start of the 1960s [5]. As a result, in sub-Saharan Africa the population received on average only 89% of the required calorie supply (1988 figures) [6].

The arrival of HIV/AIDS in a household can undermine nutritional status further, as the illness and death of one or two family members can significantly reduce food production, income and ultimately the viability of the household unit. Moreover, in many countries and particularly in Central Africa, women are the main producers of food, and since they also take on a disproportionate share of the burden of caring for those who are sick or orphaned, the amount of labour available to work the land will decline still further.

Small Farm Vulnerability

The greatest resource of small farms is their labour; they generally have few resources in terms of mechanical devices or draught-animals. Household members are often involved in both agriculture and non-farm work such as petty trading, small-scale production of goods or wage labouring. Women tend to be responsible for growing food crops and selling the surplus in local markets, as well as for the time-consuming collection of fuelwood and water. Men tend to produce the cash crops and in the dry season often migrate to earn cash income in towns and cities, returning to provide labour at critical times such as harvesting or

Credit schemes: a lifeline under threat

Credit is a tool used by governments, institutions and individuals the world over to generate income. Yet those most in need of income—the poor—are those who have least access to credit. The rural poor in particular have few or no assets to offer as security; they may not live within reach of a bank, or they may be unable to comply with the formalities of applying for a loan. And even if those hurdles are overcome, the sum they require—perhaps $100 or $50 or less to buy seed, livestock, a tool or agricultural implement—is often too small for the bank to be concerned with.

Local moneylenders will provide loans where banks do not, but at exorbitant interest rates which may draw the borrower into an ever deepening debt trap. To provide an alternative, credit schemes have emerged—some indigenous, others sponsored by international NGOs—whereby small loans are offered at reasonable rates.

To get access to credit, women often have to overcome traditional customs and practices which relegate them to inferior social, economic and political status. Some men refuse to allow their wives to obtain loans because they consider financial matters to be a male preserve or they fear their wives' financial independence. Nonetheless, women's credit schemes which have overcome these obstacles have often proved extremely successful, with women proving to be as or more reliable than men [25].

HIV/AIDS and credit schemes interact in two negative ways. Self-supporting schemes that run on narrow margins are at risk if borrowers are unable to repay loans, while raising interest rates to cover an increased number of defaulters defeats the purpose of the scheme. A real or perceived inability to repay excludes many people with HIV/AIDS from borrowing from the scheme at a time in their lives when they have most need of money. People with HIV/AIDS therefore find they either do not get access to credit in the first place, or because illness or death prevents them repaying, their assets are seized and the family ends up even worse off. Such consequences have already been observed in parts of Central Africa.

ACORD, an international NGO consortium, which sponsors several credit schemes in East Africa, has examined several means of ensuring that people with HIV/AIDS continue to have access to credit schemes. One option, of the NGO writing off loans where the borrower has died, was deemed to be impracticable because of the numbers involved. Another possibility, of lending to the family rather than an individual, is feasible in some cultures, but risks placing the main beneficiaries, particularly women, at risk. A third option is to encourage groups to discuss the possibility of death and to explore alternatives to asset seizure.

ACORD also recommends that groups reconsider the type of activities to be funded by credit in the light of HIV/AIDS. Positive contributions can be made by investing in labour-saving devices, such as a food-grinding machine or donkeys for animal traction, or income-generating activities used to fund social services, such as clinics. Projects with a quick turnover or requiring limited labour inputs should also be given priority [26].

land preparation. Cash is needed to purchase seeds and fertiliser, hire extra labour when necessary, buy food where household production provides only part of the family's requirements, and also to pay for medical expenses and social obligations [7]. As well as remittances from migrant labour, cash comes from the sale of crops, livestock and their byproducts.

Small farms are characterised by a precarious balance of income over expenditure. In Malawi, 29% of the farmholdings under 0.7 hectares consume all their food within four months of harvest and must rely on other sources of income to feed their household during the rest of the year [8]. Remittances from migrant workers are estimated to constitute between 11% and 19% of the average small (0.5-1 hectare) farmholding's total cash income [9]. Thus the loss of work in the South African mines (see pp79-80) was a significant blow to thousands of Malawians and their families. Some authorities estimate that 50% of small farms derive half their income from outside sources, a figure that rises to over 60% for households headed by women [10].

Food and Agriculture Organization (FAO) studies on Malawi and Tanzania stress the importance of remittances and seasonal labour supply, both hired and from adult male household members. The death of a male head of household from HIV/AIDS is unlikely to cause a household immediate losses in food production, but it is likely to result in loss of income. The death of a second family member, particularly a female head, is likely to affect both income and food production. Although reduced family size means lower food requirements, the remaining adults have to support an increasing number of dependants [11].

Thus smallholder agriculture in sub-Saharan Africa often operates on a fine margin of viability. This varies from district to district as farming systems are characterised by different combinations of climate, terrain, soil and crops, some more favourable than others. The demands on labour vary, with some crops being more sensitive to any interruptions. For example, a delay in maize, bean or groundnut planting substantially reduces yields. Bananas, yams and cassava, on the other hand, do not require activity at such specific periods and can be left untended for some time without affecting the harvest.

Prolonged interruption of the labour supply may also mean such vital tasks as land preparation or maintainance of irrigation systems suffer, and so in turn affect future production. Reduced cash income, if a working adult falls ill, limits the purchase of essential items such as tools, seeds and fertiliser. If the household then has to sell assets in order to meet its immediate needs, future output is also jeopardised. Some of these needs will be medical, and in areas where government health services are rudimentary, people have to resort to private medical care and so incur even greater debt; to finance this they may mortgage or sell animals or

Much African agriculture is labour-intensive and takes place on small family farms. Illness from HIV/AIDS and caring for the sick directly threatens the two most important resources of these households: their time and energy.

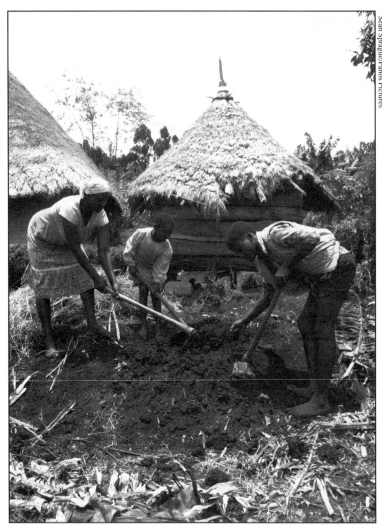

Sean Sprague/Panos Pictures

pledge future crops [12]. As the food supply suffers, so the risk of malnutrition and vulnerability to disease grows, as does the danger of being caught in the "poverty ratchet", whereby loss or sale of assets to meet short-term needs creates a cycle of impoverishment which becomes impossible to reverse.

There are useful comparisons to be made with studies on other debilitating diseases, such as river blindness and malaria. Research into the economic impact of malaria found that, because other family members increase their workload to make up for one who is sick, the household is a better unit than the individual to measure lost productivity. One of the most detailed studies shows that despite increased work by healthy members on behalf of ill ones, and extra assistance from neighbours, children and sometimes hired labour, the average reduction in the agricultural productivity of a household during a period of heavy malaria transmission can be as much as 30% [13]. However, while it is helpful to see the household as a unit of production, it is also important to recognise that within that unit, different people are affected in different ways: young girls, for example, often bear the brunt of the extra work burden and for that reason are more likely to be taken out of school.

The most vulnerable to the impact of HIV/AIDS are those households dependent on a few working adults

A 1989 study of the impact of river blindness on rural households in Guinea reveals a classic example of the "poverty ratchet". The worst effects of the disease are concentrated in "young, developing households", where a large number of dependants are supported by a small number of economically active members. Like AIDS, river blindness targets adults of working age. As the ability to produce and accumulate food and income decreases, the household falls into a downward spiral of increasing dependency ratios, poorer nutrition and health, increasing expenditure of resources (time and money) on health problems, more food shortages, decreasing household viability, and increasing reliance on support from extended family and the wider community [14].

Selective impact
The other side of this situation is that some people will benefit from others' decline. Someone will be buying up the assets that are sold, from farm implements, animals and labour to land. Thus AIDS can serve to reinforce the inequalities in a society, further widening the gap between rich and poor, although at present the evidence for this is anecdotal.

The extent to which small farms are vulnerable to HIV/AIDS depends on their ability to buy in or reallocate existing resources to compensate for lost labour and income. These resources include labour, cash reserves, household skills (including the ability to take on extra caring and parenting roles) and income-generating activities. Equally important are the social resources available: family and community networks of material and emotional support that are not easily calculated in economic analyses [15].

Richer farms, with adequate or surplus land and significant non-agricultural income, can usually afford to hire extra labour. The most vulnerable to the impact of HIV/AIDS are households dependent on a few working adults, short of land, less able to afford hired labour and with few sources of cash income. In times of need they may have to offer themselves as wage labourers to

The reality of HIV/AIDS: three households

The effect of HIV/AIDS on households is not uniform. The following case studies of real households are taken from an extensive study of the impact of the epidemic in one area of Uganda.

Household A consists of a man aged 36, a woman aged 32, their daughter of 18, and two other children aged 12 and five who are in school. There is one other younger child. They have two farm plots, a small one in their village, and another in a nearby village. It is almost certain that this man had another wife in the latter village. They grow beans, cassava, potatoes, maize, groundnuts, sorghum and bananas. They are in the process of establishing a coffee plantation in their other plot. The household employs labour for land preparation. They sell considerable amounts of their produce in the market, estimating the proportions as follows: beans 30%, maize 80%; groundnuts 30%.

Recently their teenage son died from AIDS. He was a fisherman. The husband also used to be a fisherman, then a trader; now he has turned to farming. He left the fishing to his son and ceased trading because it was unprofitable.

Because of the son's death, the household has lost a source of income. But this does not seem to have made it particularly vulnerable because there are enough resources, from some continued trading and fishing, to allow the establishment of the second farm and also to employ labour. Their teenage daughter also contributes labour, so the household has three adult workers and three dependent children. There is thus a favourable balance of consumers to workers. There are some resources to fall back on, mainly from savings and also from sales of crops. Although the death of the son has removed one income source, it has not had a profound effect on the household's ability to cope with its basic needs: the children have not been withdrawn from school. Thus the survival of this relatively rich, mature household would be threatened only by several deaths from AIDS.

Household B consists of a man aged 70, his daughter aged 30 (divorced, her children having left with her ex-husband) and a son aged 15. The man's first wife left him, as did his second wife. Two children from these marriages, a daughter aged 35 and a son aged 37, died in 1987 from AIDS.

Crops grown are coffee, bananas, cassava, potatoes, yams and beans. Their income is supplemented by smoking fish and selling it. The plot size is 0.6 hectares, not all of which is cultivated. They have plans to clear more land next season. They would like to employ additional labour but do not have enough cash.

The two adults who died from AIDS used to help on the farm. As a result of their deaths the banana farm and the annual crop land returned to bush. In addition, the 15-year-old son was taken out of school in order to help on the farm.

Thus HIV/AIDS has meant for this family that land has returned to bush and a child has been withdrawn from school. Lack of cash means that the cultivated area has effectively been reduced, but fish-processing and trading provides a minor source of additional income. This family is quite vulnerable. Were it not for the presence of the head of the family's divorced daughter (who may remarry) there would doubtless be a labour problem, given his advanced age.

Household C has suffered two deaths in the past few years. The householder's wife died from "generalised illness" and his 16-year-old daughter died of AIDS in 1988. Three people remain: the householder aged 53, a son aged 17 (who is a fisherman and does not work on the farm at all) and a daughter aged 12 (who has been withdrawn from school). They have a little land and they grow coffee, bananas and some sweet potatoes and cassava. There is not enough land to merit the employment of labourers and, in any case, they have no money to pay them.

As a result of the deaths, the man has lost his daughter's labour on potatoes and bananas, as well as his wife's work. "She was the treasurer—she always advised on questions of income and expenditure," he remarked, describing the loss of his wife's management abilities. The cropping pattern has changed. They have stopped growing groundnuts and beans (through lack of labour) and no longer maintain the bananas for the same reason. The man has to do the domestic work as well as the farming. This has meant cutting down on the time spent working the land. His relatives do not live in the village, thus they cannot help—and, he says, local people do not help non-kin.

This household has been markedly affected by the deaths, one of which was definitely from AIDS. The result has been a decreased range of crops, reduced labour inputs to the farm, withdrawal of a child from school (because of lack of cash) and loss of managerial skills and domestic labour. The son contributes some cash from his fishing but is likely to leave home shortly, thus removing a source of income. The foreseeable outcome is that this man will be left alone with his young daughter. It is unlikely that he will be able to remarry in this village, given that he is a stranger and that there has been an AIDS death in the household. It is also worth noting that he has received, and expects, little help from his extended family who live some distance away.

Tony Barnett *and* **Piers Blaikie,** *adapted from AIDS in Africa: its present and future impact, Belhaven Press, London, 1992.*

other households.

As the river blindness study showed, the age structure of the household is significant. The age of the (male or female) head of household—young (under 30), mature (30 to 55) or elderly (over 55)—usually determines the number of dependants and/or labour available. Young households with high dependency ratios will feel greater strain from the loss of an adult than mature families, although there may be cultural variations in the way households are organised, such as those run on polygamous lines, and thus in their capacity to respond to such pressures.

Agricultural Systems

Other factors affect the resilience of small farms to the AIDS epidemic. Within any country, there is likely to be a variety of farming systems supporting different kinds of crops, requiring different intensities of labour and returning different yields. A farming system with plentiful and well distributed rainfall, fertile soil and a wide range of crops will be generally less sensitive to

The primary impact of HIV/AIDS on small farms is loss of labour

labour loss than one with little rainfall, poor soils and a small range of crops, although in all systems the degree of peak labour demand remains the key factor.

An FAO study of Rwanda divided the country into five types of farming system, the most sensitive of which are based on sorghum and potato cultivation on rich volcanic soils. Less sensitive systems are based on the cultivation of beans, sweet potatoes and maize, incorporating fallow periods. The least sensitive systems are those of large landholdings where the main crops are beans, sorghum, cassava, banana and coffee. Within each system, small nuclear families were more sensitive to labour loss than larger extended ones [16].

In a typical household in the volcanic highlands of Rwanda, with a nuclear rather than extended family, women are involved in all food-related tasks (cultivation, preparation and marketing), while men are responsible for cash crops and animal husbandry. There is little migration, land is scarce, the range of crops is restricted and farming is labour-intensive [17]. Such households are particularly vulnerable to the loss of a working man, because of the high workload of women and their inability to mitigate the impact by diverting their labour.

Responses

The primary impact of HIV/AIDS on small farmholdings is loss of labour as a result of illness and death. There are various means of compensating for this loss in the short term. Those who are not ill may be able to work more hours in the day; children may be removed from school; those who can afford it can hire extra labour; and community work forces may be established at critical periods of demand or to reduce time spent on water and fuel collection. Some of these solutions are only temporary and may not be possible if many people in the household or community are affected by HIV/AIDS [18].

Another response, especially likely if there is already pressure on labour resources, is a switch to less labour-intensive crops. This is not without cost, since it may lead to poorer nutrition. The switch from legumes, such as peas, beans and pulses, to tubers, notably potatoes, cassava and sweet potatoes, involves less labour but produces less protein. Moreover, it is desirable to mix legumes and tubers since the nitrogen-fixing properties of the former increase soil fertility and so encourage the growth of the latter. If the switch is from cash crops to food crops, income will be lost. As the situation worsens, the range of crops may be

Figure 1: the impact of HIV/AIDS on small-scale agriculture

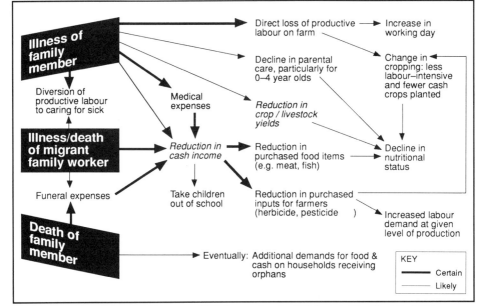

Source: Derived from diagram by T Barnett and P Blaikie reproduced in *AIDS Analysis Africa*, March/April 1991

reduced until only one staple such as bananas, which are high in carbohydrates but low in protein, or cassava, also low in protein and requiring relatively labour-intensive preparation, is grown.

Increasing productivity to compensate for lost labour can theoretically be achieved by a number of means, including the cultivation of higher yielding crops, the use of mineral fertilisers, and the mechanisation of land preparation, planting and weeding, by groups or individuals [19]. However, given the limited financial resources available to most of the affected households, such solutions are unlikely to be possible without outside assistance. High-yielding crops, for example, often need to be used in conjunction with chemical fertilisers and pesticides, so the overall investment required is considerable. There are economic implications to crop substitution at both farm and national levels. Maize, for example, needs about one-fifth of the labour required for tobacco and one-third of that required for cotton, but maize is for household consumption or local sale while tobacco and cotton are major sources of export income [20].

Poorer nutrition

In southern Uganda, household production has depended for many decades on the cultivation of *matooke* (the staple cooking banana) and of coffee as a source of cash. Good soils and plentiful

The loss of one or more working adults will gradually undermine household food security

rainfall allowed people to grow up to 12 additional crops, assuring high levels of nutrition. In some ways, HIV/AIDS is now having a more detrimental effect on this area than did the periods of war and insecurity in the 1970s and 1980s. HIV-related illness and death in many households has resulted in banana plots being tended less carefully, coffee bushes left unpruned, the size of cultivated plots being reduced and a narrower range of crops being grown. Instead of the previous wide variety of nutritious relishes, beans, peppers, potatoes and leafy vegetables, only a few remain [21]. The effects of a gradual reduction in food intake will not be immediately apparent, but are likely to lead to malnutrition.

In Rwanda the long-term effects may be increased cultivation of cassava, resorted to by many Rwandans as a famine crop, and reduced cultivation of other food and cash crops. This in turn could lead to less income from exports, and poorer nutrition. Cassava also requires more effort in preparation. Soil fertility, traditionally maintained by labour-intensive methods, may deteriorate. If the neglected land then returns to bush, there could be an increase in the numbers of tsetse flies and so in cases of sleeping sickness in humans and *ngana* in cattle [22].

Food for All

At the local level, the loss of one or more working adults from HIV/AIDS will, as the examples in this chapter show, gradually undermine household food security: the ability of the household to adequately feed all its members. But HIV/AIDS can also affect the ability of countries to feed themselves and most especially, it can threaten the ability of governments to feed their growing urban populations. First, loss of labour and so reduced food production at the local level means there is less available for consumption generally. Second, if the food producers withhold what they need for their own consumption, the fall in food availability will disproportionately affect urban dwellers, especially the poor.

Governments have two options to make up the shortfall. They can extract more food from the rural areas forcefully, as happened, for example, in the Soviet Union in the 1930s. This has the effect of transferring the famine from the politically sensitive and visible urban areas to the countryside. For all sorts of reasons, governments are unlikely to take such a course any more. The other solution is to increase food imports. This requires foreign exchange, which for most developing countries is largely generated through the export of cash crops. Most countries are already facing declining terms of trade for their exports, with every tonne of exported goods buying fewer and fewer imports.

The situation would be compounded by the fact that many smallholders might switch their own production away from cash crops to food crops, both in order to meet their own needs and because any cash crops requiring costly inputs may become beyond the reach of small farms losing labour and income because of HIV/AIDS. Moreoever, the bulk of export crops such as tea and sugar are often grown on large plantations, which rely on vast pools of low-waged labour. The advent of HIV/AIDS, besides lowering the productivity of workers, has the potential to create labour shortages for plantations, especially in the more specialised areas such as tea plucking. While detailed research on this has yet to be done, there is anecdotal evidence that in some places, such as Zaire, plantations are already beginning to face labour shortages [23].

Policies must now take into account the impact of HIV/AIDS on labour and income

Thus the time when a government may need to call on all its resources to feed its population, could be the time when it will be least able to boost local production or make up the shortfall by paying for imports from abroad.

Policy Adjustments

Rural development policy in sub-Saharan Africa must begin to consider the growing labour constraints associated with HIV/AIDS and the potential widespread disruption to the rural economy and social structure. Government policy in the past has been geared towards labour-intensive food production strategies on the basis of continued high population growth rates. In certain areas of Africa these assumptions may have to be re-examined. Policy recommendations about the relative merits of particular crops in any farming system must now take into account the impact of HIV/AIDS on labour and income. Research needs to correspond more closely to the needs of farming households with fewer working adults.

Farm support services could be strengthened to ensure that technical advice, credit and forms of labour substitution are available. The development of appropriate technologies to reduce the time spent on water and fuel collection, for example, could be critical in releasing more labour for agricultural tasks. Research into the maintenance and creation of income-generating opportunities in rural areas as alternatives to agriculture, particularly for those for whom the physical effort of farming is no longer feasible, is also essential. Finally, there may have to be

An integrated approach: Concern in Uganda

Lunyinya is a small village of 812 residents, lying between two hills in Rakai district, southwest Uganda. The brown mud houses of the village are surrounded by dark-green banana plantations. Until recently Edward Matovu lived in one of these houses, with his wife Collette and their five children, aged from 12 to two years of age.

Edward earned his meagre income from his small banana plantation. Sometimes, to supplement it, he made and sold bricks. That was until two years ago, when he started to have regular fevers and could work only occasionally on his plantation. Shortly afterwards, his wife Collette fell sick and soon they both realised they had AIDS. For the following two years it was a story of coping with the prospect of impending death while trying to live life as normally as possible and making arrangements for the children's future.

One of the first problems was a shortage of money due to reduced production and sales of crops. Members of the local Munno Mukabi group (a women's organisation, the name of which means "a friend in need") used to call round once a week to visit the family and offer what practical assistance they could. Sometimes they would tend the banana plantation. On other occasions they would draw water, collect firewood or clean the house. In order to buy medicine for himself and his wife from the local hospital, Edward sold his bicycle. As he got gradually weaker, he was forced to sell the two small pigs he possessed. Some people even sell their property in order to get money for treatment—leaving their dependants without anything following their death.

As both Edward and Collette grew gradually weaker they were no longer able to look after themselves. The burden fell on the 12-year-old daughter. After returning from school in the evening, she had to cook for the family, wash clothes and do the housework as well as her lessons—all this while watching her sick parents gradually waste away. Eventually her father withdrew her from school to help full time at home. Soon, he could no longer afford the fees, so one by one all the other three children attending school dropped out.

The local Munno Mukabi group were of some assistance to the daughter but they too were busy, trying to help nine different sick and needy people within the village. One member, Rose Bukenya, has been specially trained to care for the sick. She called round every other day in the later stages of Edward's illness. She would speak with both parents, listen to their problems, console them, and try to organise other members of Munno Mukabi to offer practical help. She would also take the Matovus for short walks when they were still able to get about.

When Edward and Collette became bedridden, Rose taught the neighbours the best way to turn them in bed, how to change sheets—sometimes soiled sheets have to be changed three times a day— and how to help them to the toilet. Before Rose taught the neighbours the most efficient way to do these things, it took four or five people instead of just two. Rose also showed the daughter the most suitable food to cook and how. The work that Rose does is voluntary.

Finally, in May 1991, Edward Matovu died, followed one month later by Collette. They are buried in simple graves beside the house, the two mounds of clay a physical reminder of their passing away.

Before Edward died, he arranged for his niece Josephine Mulindwa—who herself has two young children—to be guardian of his children. Following Collette's death, Josephine moved in. Four months later she fell sick. She, too, has AIDS.

The story of the Matovu family is a tragic drama being acted out in thousands of homes in Rakai. In 1990, 21 people died in Lunyinya village alone, mostly from AIDS. One villager has already lost nine brothers and sisters and she and her older brother are the only two remaining members of the family. In Kirumba sub-county, which includes Lunyinya, over 560 people died in 1990, mostly from AIDS. By October 1991 as many again had already died.

Building on strength

Concern is an Irish NGO working in Uganda. It is developing a number of ways to strengthen and support existing village structures and individual households as they cope with the effects of HIV/AIDS. At the individual level, the sick and their families require medicine, treatment, practical help and psychological support. Coping mechanisms often exist already. Munno Mukabi is a women's group who come together to support each other at times of need. When someone died in a village, for example, they would help cook the food for all the people coming to attend the funeral. Now, as the story of Lunyinya shows, they are increasingly involved in caring for families suffering from HIV/AIDS. Concern is helping to strengthen this voluntary society by providing training for the women in, for example, health care and running cooperatives.

By paying the fees of children pulled out of school by sick parents who can no longer afford to send them, Concern gives the children a chance of education and helps stop the slide into deeper poverty. Three of the Matovu children have returned to school under this programme. Concern workers also mobilise school children to join together once a month in community work: collecting water and firewood, cleaning houses and helping on farms.

At the village level, people's time and money is increasingly being directed towards looking after the sick. Older people are required to take on parenthood again, looking after their grandchildren. The rising number of funerals is also absorbing much time and money. One villager recalled that: "Last week I did not spend one night in my own bed at home but slept out at neighbours' houses, mourning deaths in the village."

The entrepreneurial and most educated villagers are often the first to die, depriving the community of vital skills and leadership. In Rakai district as a whole, there has been a decrease in members of the agricultural department. Since April 1991, three staff have died and at least two more are extremely ill. Only two staff have been replaced: people are reluctant to work in the region because of AIDS.

Lack of labour is the most serious economic effect of AIDS in the area. Farms are being left untended, production is dropping, and as more working adults and extension workers die, valuable agricultural skills are being lost. Some organisations are developing training courses to make sure knowledge and experience is passed on to new generations. To help raise food production and compensate for loss of labour, Concern has provided a tractor for the use of poorer families. Many widows and orphans live in households where there is no-one to till the land and so the NGO is supporting the cultivation of community plots and the creation of school farms. It has also been training local men and women in small-scale project management and simple accountancy, to help villagers diversify their farming, develop cooperatives and generate income by, for example, rearing pigs and goats. Diminishing physical energy in the sick means that people need to find less demanding ways of making a living than working the land. In addition, many women find themselves without land after the death of their husbands and so need to set up in some small trade or business.

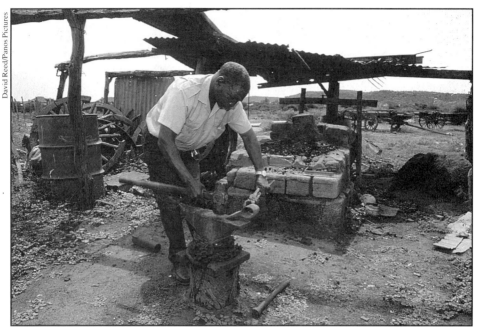

David Reed/Panos Pictures

Blacksmith, Botswana. Rural households are usually more interdependent than those in urban areas. If farmers become impoverished, so do related small businesses like this. The whole community can be caught in the "poverty ratchet".

interventions to bolster the social fabric of rural communities devastated by HIV/AIDS. Traditional household and village structures that normally play a critical role in family welfare and resource management are under strain. Research could be done into agricultural and social coping mechanisms and the experiences shared between areas with similar farming practices.

Although this chapter has of necessity concentrated on sub-Saharan Africa, many of the lessons to be learnt are relevant in other regions: only the impacts will vary, according to the different farming systems. In Asia, for example, much of which is characterised by high population density, a ready supply of landless labour and less female involvement in agriculture, some of the reactions of farming households to loss of labour will differ from those currently being observed in Africa. And there is evidence that rural areas in Asia and Latin America are increasingly being affected by HIV/AIDS, particularly through the practice of migration. One observer in Bihar, India, found that in remote villages, some 50% of the male labour force spent six months of the year working in the urban centres along the railway route to Calcutta, opening up a channel of infection right into the heartland of the rural areas. Similarly, there is a long tradition of labour migration, of men and women, in the high Andes region of Latin America, and also in Mexico [24].

CHAPTER 7

National perspectives

A decade after AIDS was first identified, economists are just beginning to take account of the impact of the epidemic on the economies of the most affected countries. Economic policies have tended to be based on the assumption that labour will not be a constraint to development, yet it is clear that in these countries HIV/AIDS has the potential to lower productivity and reduce the supply of skilled and experienced workers. In some areas, there has been a loss of unskilled labour as well—the potential disruption to food supplies has already been discussed. But the epidemic is likely to affect every sector of the economy and countries which are dependent on a few key industries or sectors are particularly vulnerable.

For many developing countries, the HIV/AIDS epidemic has emerged in the context of a decade of economic recession, worsening climatic and environmental problems, and social unrest. Since the early 1980s, per capita incomes have risen in much of Asia; in contrast they have fallen, in some cases drastically, in many parts of Africa and Latin America. Unfavourable terms of trade are a factor in this decline. In Africa, on a per capita basis, the real purchasing power of exports in 1990 was about one-third of what it was 10 years earlier [1]. Of the 42 nations known as the Least Developed Countries (LDCs), a term which includes social as well as economic indicators of poverty, 29 are in Africa; Asia and the Pacific have 12 and Latin America one. The number of African LDCs may increase as more countries apply to be included.

In sub-Saharan Africa, where the impact of HIV/AIDS is currently greatest, many economies are already in decline—in itself, a factor in the spread of the disease. These economies face further loss of productivity as the burden of the epidemic spreads beyond the individual and the household, to the fields, factories and offices, and then to the national economy; investment in both human and physical capital is threatened, while financial services are directly influenced by dwindling national and household savings. In the worst-affected countries, key services like electricity generation, transport, health, housing, and the armed forces and police may be affected by skilled labour shortages.

Those countries of Latin America, the Caribbean and Asia which have richer and more diverse economies are less at risk; nevertheless, they remain vulnerable to an increasing burden from the epidemic on the supply of labour, investment and ultimately their prospects of development.

For governments and business, the growing costs associated with widespread HIV infection in the labour force could reduce levels of savings and investment and frustrate aspirations of economic growth. If key exports fall, access to foreign exchange will become more difficult, limiting a country's ability to import goods and services and pay interest on its foreign debt. Foreign investment may be withheld if economic prospects suggest little return, while greater dependency on foreign aid may not be matched by greater infusions of money from donor countries.

The Importance of Skilled Labour

At first glance, predicting shortages in the labour supply as a result of HIV/AIDS may be hard to reconcile with existing high levels of unemployment and underemployment. It is, however, the lack of skills and education, together with shortages of investment capital and foreign exchange, which underlie persistent underemployment in many countries. As HIV/AIDS has a disproportionate impact on the skilled labour force, this only exacerbates the problem. Moreover, if the potential losses in the informal sector (subsistence farming, small-scale business and industry) and of women's unpaid labour are added to the losses in the cash economy, it is clear that the impact on the national economy can become severe indeed.

Industries or commercial enterprises which are heavily dependent on skilled labour are more sensitive to the epidemic. In Zambia, copper mining yields over 75% of export earnings and produces more than a quarter of the gross national product (GNP). Although the industry employs only 6% of the country's labour force, about one-third of the employees are skilled: equipment operators, mining engineers, managers, accountants and others. Thus a key component of the country's economy is dependent on a small group of highly trained and experienced workers, who are difficult to replace either from within the country, or by employing expatriates, because the cost of the latter is prohibitive within the narrow profit margins essential for export markets.

In countries where the key industry is likely to be seriously affected—to the point where it would no longer be internationally competitive—policymakers will have to make some difficult choices over strategies and priorities. Faced with a serious decline in critical export earnings, they may be forced—at least in the short term—to consider concentrating whatever resources are available to limit the impact of the disease, on the workforce in this key industry. More comprehensive policies may have to wait.

Enterprises heavily dependent on skilled labour are more sensitive to the epidemic

Mike Bailey, a specialist on HIV/AIDS and development who has worked with UNDP, points to the other potential implications of the epidemic in countries dependent on the expertise of a small group of skilled people: "Take, for example, a landlocked country with a small national airline. What happens when the pilots or engineers fall ill and cannot be replaced? That's a significant blow to the country's independence and prestige. Or what about a country dependent on irrigation where there is just a handful of hydrologists [2]?" Table 3 in Chapter 5 gives some idea of the narrow skill base in some countries.

In addition, there is a knock-on effect in other sectors of an economy when one component is adversely affected. For example, whatever their skill base, commercial enterprises for a mainly local market may be affected by a fall in demand for their products or services, as consumers become poorer and allocate more of their income to expenditure on medical and other costs associated with HIV/AIDS.

Savings

By reducing productivity, HIV/AIDS reduces income, which has an impact on savings at all levels of the economy. The quantity of savings available and how they are used are key factors which determine an economy's rate of growth.

In much of the South, and particularly in sub-Saharan Africa, government savings play a critical role in providing social welfare programmes and in investment in infrastructure and production. As the costs of HIV/AIDS prevention and medical care rise, there will be increased pressure for spending on health care. At the same time, the threat to skilled labour will make governments reluctant to divert funds from education.

With few opportunities to increase revenue through taxation and with export income likely to remain low as a result of depressed commodity prices, funds may be diverted from capital investment and maintenance of infrastructure. Maintaining existing spending priorities through borrowing or inflationary finances remains a limited option, given the already unsustainable

Zimbabwe

Zimbabwe is a landlocked Southern African country inhabited by nearly 10 million people. Seventy-two per cent of the population lives in rural areas. Since becoming independent in 1980, Zimbabwe has had mixed economic success. In 1992 it faced two major crises: in the short term an exceptionally severe drought, and in the long term the potentially devasting spread of HIV/AIDS.

The incidence of HIV is relatively high, reaching 18% in the capital, Harare. It is generally believed that the virus will continue to spread despite efforts at education and condom provision. Although there are currently no data on the rate of spread, there have been various attempts to model the progress of the epidemic. It is clear that the disease will not cause the population of Zimbabwe to drop in the foreseeable future. This means that the country will not face an overall labour shortage but, as in most African countries, there is a surplus of unskilled and semi-skilled labour. It is the impact on the limited pool of skilled, professional staff which will have the most effect on the economy.

By African standards the Zimbabwean economy is well developed. In 1989, it had a per capita GDP of $640, the ninth highest in sub-Saharan Africa, although over the last decade economic performance has been erratic. Manufacturing and agriculture are the most important productive sectors. The size of the manufacturing sector, which provides over 25% of GDP, is an indication of the maturity of the Zimbabwean economy [14].

Agriculture provides a quarter of formal sector employment; the bulk of the exports; inputs for industry; and is the major source of food and income for millions of subsistence farmers. In general the country is self-sufficient in food, and in good years exports maize and wheat. Unfortunately the 1991/92 growing season saw the worst drought for decades. It is estimated that that 1 million tonnes of maize and 250,000 tonnes of wheat will have been imported, and 2 million people will have required food aid. There are predictions that Zimbabwe's GDP will fall by 3% in 1992 as a result of the drought [15].

The drought is likely to fuel the spread of HIV by giving impetus to rural-urban migration, increasing the levels of malnutrition and poverty, and provoking massive social dislocation. In turn, HIV/AIDS may affect the agricultural sector. Commercial agriculture contributes significantly to the economy and provides both food and export crops, mainly tobacco and cotton. The·Commercial Farmers Union (CFU) was one of the first groups to introduce HIV/AIDS education, yet they have already begun to experience a loss of labour as a result of the epidemic and are warning of the economic and social costs [16].

The deaths of skilled and experienced staff will have a damaging and, in the short term, unquantifiable effect on the operations of the private sector parastatals and the government. Some companies have been quick to react, introducing HIV/AIDS education for their workers. Other responses include increasing the level of training in order to provide for anticipated deaths from AIDS; in some cases, the number of trainees has been doubled. Some companies have introduced pre-employment screening, thus restricting employment opportunities for people who may have years of productive life left.

Zimbabwe is unique among African countries in that it has a developed private medical sector with medical aid schemes. The current average cost per AIDS case to these schemes is estimated at Z$4,000 ($800). The medical societies warn that treating AIDS could be an insupportable burden to the private schemes, although they cannot morally or practically avoid the costs of people with HIV/AIDS [17].

The state has not attempted to assess the cost of HIV-related disease to the health care

sector, but it is known to be large and growing, and an increasing number of hospital beds are occupied by HIV/AIDS patients. The health sector was one of the successes of Zimbabwe in the post-independence period: infant mortality fell from 86 to 61 per 1,000 births and life expectancy increased from 55 to 59 years. These gains are under attack from both the growing HIV/AIDS epidemic and the structural adjustment package which the government has adopted.
Alan Whiteside, *Economic Research Unit, University of Natal, South Africa*

burdens of public debt servicing and the pressure from international institutions such as the International Monetary Fund (IMF) to control spending as a condition for continued loans or investment. Over the medium to long term, a further reduction in government savings and investment is the likely outcome.

As companies have to spend more and more on provision for HIV/AIDS, for example increasing training programmes and revising pension, sickness benefit and insurance schemes, so their profits will be reduced. This will affect their ability to invest and thus have a long-term impact on the economy.

In many developing countries, household income is supplemented by remittances from family members working abroad. These remittances are increasingly included in government calculations of economic performance and outlook. In some countries they follow exports as the second most important source of foreign exchange earnings and thus comprise a critical source of national savings. This traditional safety net is threatened if foreign governments or corporations discriminate against labour from countries with high HIV infection rates. Thailand's dependence on foreign remittances has already been noted—migrant workers sent home nearly $1 billion in 1991—while Malawi recently lost $27 million a year after the Malawian government prevented its nationals from working in South African mines as a protest against their policy of testing workers for HIV [3]. In 1991, Johann Liebenberg of the South African Chamber of Mines was quoted as saying that as a result of pre-employment testing and the Malawian government's reaction to it, only 36 Malawians were working in the industry [4], compared to an estimated 20,000 five years earlier.

Foreign aid
Faced with the financial constraints associated with structural adjustment programmes and the impact of HIV/AIDS, developing countries may become increasingly reliant on foreign aid to sustain social welfare programmes and to underwrite development efforts. Yet these sources of finance are shrinking.

Losses from HIV/AIDS could be more than offset by improved policies in the next decade

For example, Official Development Assistance (ODA)—which takes the form of grants from governments and UN agencies as well as low interest loans—for Africa has remained static since 1986 at about $20 billion annually (despite a population increase of approximately 9%), while for developing countries as a whole it fell from $58 billion in 1985 to $54 billion in 1990 [5].

The prospects look even grimmer within the context of the new global competition for capital. According to an analysis by the Organisation for Economic Co-operation and Development (OECD)—a grouping of industrialised countries—the predicted stagnation in development loans and grants reflects a worldwide shortage of capital, which itself stems from declining national savings performance in the OECD countries since 1984 [6]. This decline has been partly aggravated by the new set of demands for aid arising out of the wave of political and economic liberalisation in Central and Eastern Europe and the former USSR.

The new competition for capital is reflected in donors' increasing concern with the effectiveness of their contributions; there is closer scrutiny by donors and international lending agencies of the economic and social policies of recipient countries and the strings attached to loans are increasing in number and stringency. It is not yet clear to what extent these agencies will take into consideration the economic impact of the HIV/AIDS epidemic in their calculations of performance targets, which are built into their conditions for continued support of developing countries.

Foreign investment

Foreign investment plays varying roles in the South. Although it forms a relatively substantial source of additional savings in Asia and Latin America, it is almost negligible in sub-Saharan Africa, in itself a major hindrance to the region's development prospects. HIV/AIDS may become a deterrent to foreign investment in seriously affected countries as foreign investors perceive the epidemic disrupting labour markets. While a multinational company such as Unilever will consider "political risk a more serious factor than AIDS in determining investment [7]", the epidemic is itself a factor increasing the level of economic and therefore social instability in badly affected countries. Lower levels of investment will mean less productive employment, lower income and slower rates of economic growth.

The Thai study reports that a large supply of inexpensive labour is a key attraction for foreign businesses investing in Thailand. "Foreign direct investment has surpassed $2 billion

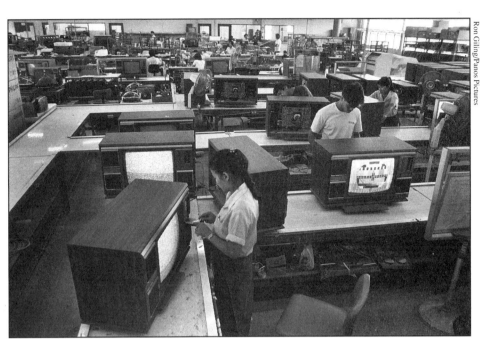

annually for the past two years. A reduction in the supply and health of labour could increase both wage rates and production costs, making Thailand a less attractive place to invest in [8]."

Studies have been done to examine the implications for specific countries in more detail (see Box overleaf). The Thai study predicts that unless significant behaviour change occurs, the HIV/AIDS epidemic is likely to alter the performance of the country's economy, which grew at an average of 4.5% per year throughout the 1980s [9].

Philips electronics factory, near Bangkok. "A reduction in the supply and health of labour could... make Thailand a less attractive place to invest in."

Economic Strategies

It is too early to tell whether the predictions of the economic models described overleaf will be realised, but once they are, it will be too late to take preventive action. This does mean, however, that there is time to intervene to slow the spread of the disease and to make the economy more resistant in the longer term. Losses resulting from HIV/AIDS could be more than offset by improved policies in the next decade. Countries where levels of infection appear much lower, such as China and the new republics of the former USSR, have the best chance of preventing an epidemic, although success will be limited if there is not the political will to take account of the social and economic aspects of the epidemic, rather than just the medical ones.

The cost of lost lives

Chapter 3 discussed the **direct** (medical) costs of HIV/AIDS; **indirect** costs are an attempt to measure the costs of illness and death of adults of working age in terms of their lost income. Indirect costs are generally calculated by estimating the number of years of working life and potential earnings lost by a person acquiring the disease. There are many problems in valuing present labour time; placing a value on future labour is even more difficult. To do so, health economists frequently use average urban wages and assume that the value of labour does not change over time.

As with the mathematical models predicting the demographic impacts (see Chapter 2), models of the economic impact are more valuable for the understanding they offer of how the epidemic affects the economy, than as absolute predictions of the future. They can be varied to include different levels of productivity and income, as a result of differing education, skill or age. Models may also approximate the losses which occur if other workers' productivity is lost, through time spent caring for the ill or because of disruptions to production caused by labour shortages or reduced investment. Other variables include assumptions about how many people are infected, their age, the incubation period of the disease, replacement costs and the age at which individuals enter and leave the workforce. Few models include the labour which is outside the cash economy but is nevertheless essential to economic survival, such as women's labour in the household or food production, children's labour in collecting fuel and water, and reciprocal or communal labour schemes within communities during times of peak demand. The loss of any of these directly affects an individual's or a household's standards of living. Nor do economic models take into account the informal economy—market trading, small-scale business and industry—which in some areas provides employment for up to 70% of the population. Thus extrapolating the economic costs of HIV to a nation's population on the basis of urban incomes is likely to distort the reality, especially as the epidemic spreads from higher to lower socio-economic groups and from urban centres to rural communities.

Even greater uncertainty is involved in projecting future changes and incorporating factors which are indirectly related or unrelated to HIV/AIDS, such as terms of trade, changing interest and wage rates, and levels of savings, all of which can greatly influence national economic performance. Any estimate of the indirect costs of the epidemic should therefore be treated with circumspection, because it refers only to one possible scenario of many.

A 1988 World Bank study of the costs of HIV infection in Tanzania and Zaire estimated annual indirect costs for people who died of AIDS as between $890 and $2,663 in Zaire and between $2,425 and $5,093 in Tanzania (1985 figures); variations reflected different educational backgrounds. The figures assumed an average of 8.8 healthy life years lost and assigned different productivity losses according to age. When the direct (medical) costs were included, total annual costs per person ranged from 15-54 times per capita GDP in Zaire and 24-52 times per capita GDP in Tanzania [10].

Another study based on the same information estimated the overall cost to these two countries of HIV/AIDS. It assumed that if all those who developed AIDS were in work and had an average income of urban workers with a primary school education, an HIV/AIDS incidence of 0.5% would mean a permanent reduction in gross national product (GNP) of 0.8% in Tanzania and 1% in Zaire. If the concentration of cases in the largest cities meant that the average income of people with HIV/AIDS was that of urban workers with secondary school incomes, the same incidence would result in direct labour productivity costs of 1.5%-2% of GNP. If medical costs and withdrawals from the labour market to help take care of the ill were included, these figures might double [11].

In Thailand, working on the basis that a person with HIV/AIDS has an average annual income of $1,500 and that their death results in the loss of 25 years of working life, lost earnings average over $22,000 per death. This figure reflects the "discounting of prime adult years": a statistical method that assumes future life is less valuable than present life. By including annual health care costs of $615-$1,000 per year, total costs are equal to 16-18 times per capita GDP. For the country as a whole, total annual health care costs plus value of lost income is projected to grow from $100 million in 1991 to $1.8 billion-$2.2 billion by 2000. Over these 10 years, between $7.3 and $8.7 billion will be lost due to HIV/AIDS-related illness and death [12].

In a 1988 study, the economic value of a year of prime life in Puerto Rico was determined at $5,700. The island's minimum wage was used as an estimate of average earnings and the island's high unemployment was taken into account. Assuming 13.29 prime working years lost per adult case, the value of the indirect costs per case is $80,000. Including direct costs of $22,541 per case, total costs per case are 19 times per capita GDP. Based on the numbers of cases reported, total costs were estimated as $100 million—0.54% of the island's GDP. By 1992, the study projected, costs would rise to $541.2 million or 2.6% of current GDP [13].

It must always be borne in mind, however, that these figures are based on a set of assumptions that work towards making the resulting costs high rather than low. For example, different assumptions about average earnings (the rural majority might well earn less than the minimum wage) could lead to very different figures.

Even though the predictions of the likely costs of the epidemic can be no more than speculative, they provide a tool with which to lobby government leaders and policymakers, and they help draw national attention to the epidemic, and encourage effective and immediate action to reduce its spread. The scenarios of cascading losses can, however, lead to a paralysing pessimism. Nevertheless, the suggestion that portions of Africa and Asia may have to be "written off", as rates of infection reach levels which threaten to cause social and economic collapse, should be rejected on both humanitarian and factual grounds. While the economic losses are potentially large, they are still far less than the damage to economies which stems from, for example, prolonged drought, declining export prices and political unrest. And as the next chapter makes clear, spending on HIV/AIDS prevention and education activities now, pays huge dividends in terms of saving far higher economic costs later.

In areas where labour, particularly skilled labour, becomes a constraint for the first time, there will be an urgent need for labour-saving appropriate technologies to maintain production in both agriculture and industry. To meet future demands, present initiatives to develop human resources need to be strengthened.

Nepal

Already close to the bottom of the global scale in terms of social, economic and health indicators, Nepal would find a severe HIV/AIDS epidemic devastating. And yet the conditions that facilitate the spread of HIV/AIDS—poverty and migration—are all widespread in the country.

Among the most striking aspects of Nepal's confrontation with the epidemic are the lack of data and the almost complete inability of the government to tackle the problem. Political unrest since late 1989 and the preoccupations of a newly established democracy have affected AIDS activities as much as they have other programmes. Voluntary agencies have only just begun to function and are not yet geared to tackle the task of HIV/AIDS prevention and control. The incidence of HIV/AIDS and its contribution to levels of illness and death are difficult to assess in the absence of reliable surveillance data, which is compounded by the lack of diagnostic facilities.

Nepal, with a population of 19.1 million, has a per capita GNP of $180. In the Human Development Index, Nepal ranks 140 out of 160 developing countries, with life expectancy at birth being 52.2 years and an adult literacy rate of 25.6%. Twelve million Nepalis do not have access to safe drinking water, while 18 million do not have access to sanitation. Nearly 12 million live below the poverty line.

Health indicators are abysmally bleak. According to 1990 figures, only 6% of births are attended by health personnel and infant mortality is 123 per 1,000 live births. Maternal mortality is 850 per 100,000. Nepal is one of the few countries where life expectancy for women is less than that for men. There is on average one nurse per 4,680 people and one doctor per 32,710, but half the doctors and health facilities are concentrated in the Kathmandu valley, where under 5% of the population lives. Only 5.5% of the national budget (about $27 million) is spent on health, representing an average annual per capita expenditure of $1.50. Infectious and parasitic diseases are the prime killers.

Nepal's economic base is limited: agriculture accounts for over half the country's GDP and employs over 90% of the labour force. Tourism provides about 20% of the country's earnings and industry accounts for 14% of GDP. Exploitable natural resources apart from hydro power are limited. Physical strength and youth are the only assets available to much of the country's population. Many work in traditionally underpaid and exploitative areas of manual labour, including carpet-weaving. Many Nepalis earn very little and there is severe unemployment. Over 40% of the population is underemployed.

An epidemic begins

The first recorded cases of AIDS in Nepal were in 1986 among Western tourists and Nepali women returning from brothels in Indian cities. By early 1992, there were 52 recorded cases and the male to female ratio was almost 1:1, which suggests that transmissions have taken place between couples within the country. However, extrapolating from these data is unsatisfactory because they are based on so small a sample.

The major source of HIV entry into the country is via the more than 100,000 Nepali women working in Indian brothels. Poverty is so deep and employment opportunities so limited in some of Nepal's hill areas, that it has become common practice for young women to spend some time earning money as prostitutes in India. When they return, many are accepted back into their communities, marry and have families of their own. In Bombay alone, there are estimated to be 45,000 Nepalis, some 45% of the city's sex workers.

According to the Indian Health Organisation, 30% of brothel workers in Bombay are HIV-positive. If infection rates of sex workers in other Indian cities are similar to those in Bombay, up to 30,000 Nepali women may be infected. Brothel keepers, health authorities and the police in India deport sex workers found to be HIV-positive. This means many thousands of infected women return to Nepal, where their families must take on the burden of caring for them. In addition, some of the many women who return voluntarily are likely to be infected but unaware of their HIV status.

A second group at risk is the 300,000 migrant labourers, mostly male, who have traditionally sought seasonal employment in urban centres throughout India. Migrant workers have always brought back STDs to the Nepali hills—they are known as "Bombay diseases"—and there is no doubt that HIV has joined the list of such diseases.

A third but relatively minor source of transmission is through businessmen travelling to Bangkok and other cities, as well as those engaged as couriers in the lucrative smuggling trade with Southeast Asia.

While WHO and other international agencies, particularly UNDP, are aware that the government has neither the staff nor the means to prevent the epidemic, they have so far been unable to work together and develop a comprehensive programme to contain the situation and prevent it spiralling out of control. None of the population groups most at risk have been reached with information and there is no sustained public education programme.

During 1991 and 1992 there has been the sporadic airing of a radio drama and a televised serial dealing with HIV/AIDS, but those most at risk of HIV infection are the poorest of the poor, living in remote, inaccessible hills, where there is no television, radio reception is poor and literacy levels are low. Yet it is in these hill areas that the warning signs are increasingly being picked up that an epidemic is beginning.

Thus in Nepal, because HIV/AIDS is predominantly entering communities through women returning from Indian brothels, it will strike the rural poor first and then move into the cities. The labour of the rural poor is hard to quantify economically; but while the loss of 25-30 years of productive life may not seem significant in financial terms, it is devastating to the families who depend on it. The pattern of transmission in Nepal may mean that the impact remains "invisible" for some time, and that only when the formal economy begins to suffer and the skilled and educated begin to be hit by the disease, will official action will be taken—which will be a tragedy for the country and its people.

Shanta Basnet Dixit, *Kathmandu*

Any delays will magnify future shortages and as a result increase the impact of the epidemic on economic growth rates. By the time a critical infection level in a given sector is reached or surpassed, it will be hard to make effective policy decisions.

Economic strategies, then, which take realistic account of the likely effects of the epidemic can have a measured effect in containing, and so minimising, the consequences. Efforts to promote rural development and curb urban unemployment may also help. Successful rural development policies could help slow down the pace of urbanisation and the increased migration taking place in many parts of the developing world, both processes

The Dominican Republic

The HIV/AIDS epidemic has been recognised as present in the Caribbean for some 10 years. Migration between islands and to the mainland, usually the United States, as well as drug use and, in some areas, sex tourism are all factors which facilitate transmission in the region. Levels of infection vary and some countries are severely affected. These include Haiti, which shares the island of Hispaniola with the Dominican Republic, although cultural differences mean there is little intermingling between the two peoples. The Dominican Republic faces an uncertain future as far as HIV/AIDS is concerned, but it has many of the social and economic conditions which make people vulnerable to the epidemic. Currently, 40,000-60,000 people (about 1% of the country's adult population) are estimated to have contracted the virus, but high levels of poverty and illiteracy and low levels of access to health care place many people at risk. The situation is exacerbated by the fact that only 1% of GNP is designated for health, and half of that goes on wages. According to Rita Mena Peguerro, an economist from Fundacion Economia y Desarrollo, there have been no official attempts to study any possible economic impact of the disease. Poverty is widespread. The poorest 20% of the population receives 2.66% of the total income, while the richest 20% receives 60.7%. More than 2 million people are illiterate; 1.4 million have no access to health services; 2.7 million are without clean drinking water; and 2.8 million do not have access to any sanitary services. For many of these people, HIV/AIDS is just another problem, way down on their list of priorities.

The country's financial base is broad but relatively weak. The main sources of income are trade (26.3%), industry (14.5%); and agriculture and livestock (13.1%). Some 14% of the labour force is unemployed. Small businesses generate most employment opportunities and the informal sector contributes 23% of GDP. Economic sectors potentially at risk from a worsening epidemic include the free trade zones and industrial parks, although some consider that with existing levels of unemployment there will always be people to replace those unable to work. Tourism, responsible for 39% of the country's foreign income, is very susceptible to the impact of the epidemic. As a service industry employing many people, it could be adversely affected by labour shortages. In addition, it attracts some tourists because of a large, internationally-orientated sex industry, which might be seen as a potential source of infection. A fall in the number of tourists visiting Haiti in the early 1980s was partly attributed to this cause [18].

Although the epidemic remains under the surface in the Dominican Republic, there are many tragic examples of its impact. Take the case of Pedro, a brilliant agricultural engineer who received a scholarship to study abroad. Just before concluding his course, he had to return home for special care for a bad case of pneumonia. Six months later he was dead from AIDS, leaving his family both emotionally and financially drained. The cost to the country of these untimely deaths of qualified personnel is steadily growing.

Some well-structured prevention programmes have succeeded in informing people about HIV/AIDS and have developed activities for specific population groups. Nonetheless, it is clear that the majority of the population is not aware of the dimensions of the problem, and what is more worrying, nor are the politicians. "We need more political will from the government. Specific measures have to be taken, such as increasing the funds for prevention programmes. We need more help from the media, more commitment from the business sector," says Santos Rosario, a director of a leading HIV/AIDS organisation.

Martha Butler de Lister, *Santo Domingo*

The potential to respond to HIV

The less money available to support prevention measures to limit the spread of HIV, the greater the likely impact of the epidemic. The following chart is a crude estimate of the potential ability of different countries to respond to the pandemic, drawn up by comparing the severity of the epidemic in different countries with the resources available.

Taking the United States as a baseline, the chart compares the wealth of 14 countries with the estimated proportion of each country's population infected with HIV. Column one gives an estimate of the proportion of the population which is HIV-positive. Column two shows that infection rate as a percentage of the US infection rate: the higher the number, the worse the epidemic. Column three shows GNP per capita expressed as a percentage of US GNP per capita.

The final column is an HIV resources index: per capita GNP divided by the scale of the epidemic (column three as a percentage of column two). Countries with an index of over 100 are currently better placed than the United States to respond to HIV/AIDS. Smaller indices reflect a worse position.

HIV resources index

	HIV cases per million people*	HIV epidemic index	GNP per capita as % of US**	HIV resources index
Sweden	1,000	17	71	417
Switzerland	3,636	60	89	148
France	3,565	59	68	115
USA	**6,019**	**100**	**100**	**100**
Mexico	1,000	17	10	59
Trinidad & Tobago	2,500	42	15	36
India	469	8	2	25
Brazil	4,654	77	12	16
Thailand	5,386	89	6	7
Dominican Republic	7,000	116	4	3
Kenya	7,450	124	2	2
Zimbabwe	50,000	831	3	0.4
Zaire	20,000	332	1	0.3
Rwanda	50,000	831	2	0.2
Uganda	69,149	1,149	1	0.1

* Population figures calculated from data in *Human Development Report 1992*, UNDP, and estimates of HIV infection taken from various sources
** Calculated from data in *World Development Report 1991*, World Bank

The index takes no account of actual spending priorities. The broad conclusion to be drawn, however, is that the developing world is at a severe economic disadvantage in dealing with the HIV/AIDS epidemic, with the United States having a hundred to a thousand times the economic resources to deal with the disease than the four worst-placed countries in the list.

A car factory in Trinidad. Key businesses and industries need to adopt HIV/AIDS policies before it is too late to take preventive action. Education now saves major economic costs later.

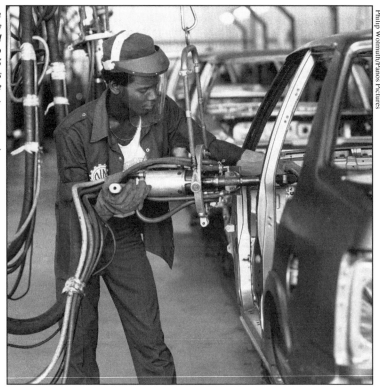

which assist HIV/AIDS transmission. Policies that promote a better standard of living for the poor and which in particular increase economic opportunities and independence for women, also help to address some of the basic inequalities which increase people's vulnerability to HIV/AIDS. Clearly both public health and economic measures are needed; neither can work in isolation. If behavioural change is achieved, it will reduce the rate of transmission of the disease and substantially lower the economic costs of the epidemic—the next chapter looks at education and prevention programmes, and examines their costs and effectiveness.

CHAPTER 8

Containing the epidemic

As the previous chapters demonstrate, HIV/AIDS has the capacity to seriously undermine the development prospects of many nations. In the worst-hit areas of Africa, it has already exacted a heavy human and economic toll. Yet despite the obvious savings to be generated by programmes to reduce the spread of HIV, actual spending is far lower than required. WHO estimates that in the developing world $0.46 is spent per person per year on all HIV/AIDS-related activities (including training, blood screening, education, care and counselling) approved by National AIDS Control Programmes (NACPs) [1]. Even if an equivalent amount is being spent on HIV/AIDS prevention by organisations outside the NACPs, still less than $1 per person per year is being spent on all HIV/AIDS activities in the developing world.

One of the main reasons for this is the long incubation period of the virus, which hides the real cost until the disease is well established. This means that the most effective interventions require the commitment and spending of funds at a time when their benefit remains theoretical. Governments worldwide are notorious for avoiding this kind of issue. The situation is further complicated by the fact that, while most health problems are linked to social and economic factors, in the case of HIV/AIDS the correlation with poverty and disadvantage is particularly intricate. This, combined with the fact that it is predominantly transmitted by sexual intercourse, means that programmes to contain it are more complex and wide-ranging than for many other diseases. Behaviour change is the key to containing the epidemic, and this is circumscribed by the social and economic circumstances of people's lives.

The mathematical models examined in Chapter 2, which gave some different scenarios for reducing the scale of the pandemic, all demonstrate that the effectiveness of interventions (actions to reduce the spread of HIV) depends to a great extent on the point in the history of the epidemic at which they are introduced. As

Proportional cost of delaying the start of an effective HIV programme

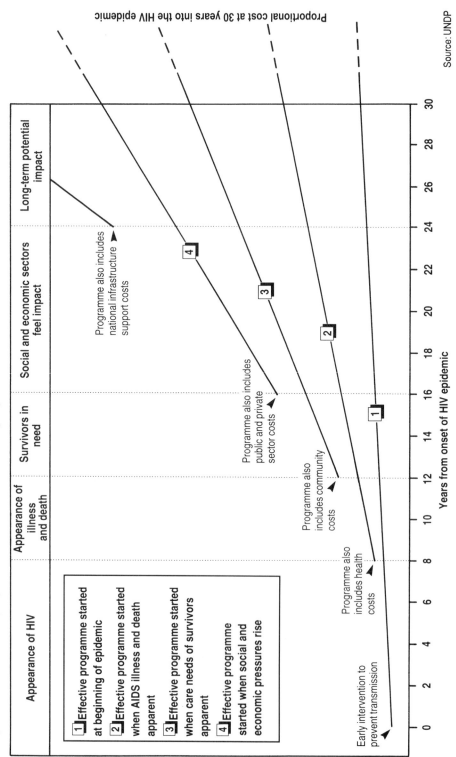

Source: UNDP

the chart opposite shows, enormous benefits are gained by reducing the heterosexual transmission of HIV infection as soon as possible. As the epidemic takes hold, the costs spread from being mainly the cost of medical care and treatment, to the longer-term costs of falling productivity and loss of skilled labour, first at the community and then at the national level. Any delay significantly increases the demographic, economic and social consequences of the epidemic.

Less than $1 per person per year is spent on HIV/AIDS activities in the developing world

Countries with low or negligible rates of infection, such as the republics of the former USSR, have most to gain from implementing intervention programmes before HIV infection becomes widespread or cases of AIDS appear. Roy Anderson emphasises the point: "Even when levels of HIV infection are low in the general population and AIDS is not the leading cause of adult and infant mortality in countries afflicted by many other serious diseases, significant resources should be directed towards inducing behavioural changes to try to prevent a widely disseminated lethal epidemic in 10 to 20 years' time [2]."

Interventions

Actions taken to reduce the spread of HIV include ensuring that blood products are screened and syringes are sterilised (see Box overleaf). These are relatively straightforward interventions. Far more complex is the prevention of transmission through sexual intercourse—through decreased numbers of partners, increased use of condoms and reduction of the incidence of STDs. Heterosexual intercourse accounts for over 75% of existing global infection and up to 90% in developing countries. Because the potential for transmission of the virus through other means is limited, the greatest impact on the future course of the epidemic will thus be through interventions in an area of human activity which is one of the most private and sensitive, yet which reflects wider social and cultural norms.

It has occasionally been argued that the best means to prevent transmission of HIV through sexual intercourse or drug injection is to identify and isolate all those known to be carrying the virus. As well as being ethically unacceptable, experience in many countries has shown that such measures are at best ineffective and at worst likely to lead to further spread of the virus, not least because they encourage people to deny the problem exists. As long as a vaccine is unavailable, only voluntary behaviour change will lead to a containment of the epidemic [3].

Interventions

Interventions can reduce transmission of HIV in every setting, except from mother to infant.

Technically, the easiest intervention is blood screening. This has been the first priority of many health authorities and funding agencies. Since infected blood is responsible for only a small percentage of transmission—no more than 10% in even the worst-affected countries—blood screening has a relatively small impact on the epidemic. Although the proportion is small, in Africa the numbers are not inconsiderable, because blood transfusions are relatively common for women and children (because of the high incidence of anaemia and birth complications); and members of the family are often the blood donors. It has been argued that the cost of universal screening is too high for many developing countries [46], while lack of resources and weak infrastructure prevent many hospitals and clinics from maintaining a steady supply of screened blood [47]. However, others have claimed that blood screening is cost-effective if rates of infection are 0.3% or higher [48].

Transmission of HIV in Romania and the former USSR show that localised epidemics from the medical use of non-sterile needles are possible. However, these form a very small proportion of cases and, through the adoption of adequate sterilisation techniques or provision of single-use syringes, are relatively simple to prevent.

Countries as diverse as Italy, Thailand and the United States demonstrate the rapidity with which HIV can spread through shared needles in injecting drug use. But as a proportion of actual cases—an estimated 5%-10% of global HIV infection—and potential cases, injecting drug users form no more than an estimated 0.3% of the world population [49], and so this form of transmission is also relatively small. Information programmes complemented by the provision of sterile syringes through needle-exchange schemes have drastically reduced the impact of the epidemic in such groups.

Behaviour Change

Gay men in many countries of the industrialised world have modified their sexual behaviour as a result of HIV/AIDS. The rate of homosexual transmission has fallen significantly since interventions by non-government organisations (NGOs) began in the early 1980s. In the United States, for example, the incidence of HIV infection has decreased significantly since the 1980s [4]. Severe epidemics in the gay populations of Northern Europe, Canada and Australia appear to have been averted because most homosexual men in these countries have followed the example of their US counterparts.

However, such success is extremely patchy and has not been easily repeated in other population groups. Indeed, a feature of many AIDS conferences has been the frequency with which some delegates report that populations most at risk, even in the worst affected areas, are continuing to have many sexual partners without using condoms [5]. Consultant sociologist Rebecca Nyonyintono reported at a seminar in Kampala in 1991 that in parts of Uganda "many are overwhelmed by the burden of care for the orphans and their own children under the commonly-practised African extended family system. But they are not taking action to prevent the spread of AIDS by modifying their own sexual behaviour [6]." A similar lack of response has been seen in the United States, where it has been pointed out that African American teenagers have a high awareness of AIDS but seldom take measures to protect themselves from HIV [7]. The UK Health Education Authority also reports that while high levels of knowledge and awareness about HIV/AIDS and condom protection have been reached within a relatively short period, any sustained shift in behaviour change among heterosexuals has yet to be achieved [8].

Information on HIV/AIDS needs to be culturally appropriate

This is not as baffling as it may at first seem. Many people persist in unhealthy activities, such as smoking, even when they are aware of the need to change and have the ability to do so. There is often a highly subjective element in people's attitudes to risk-taking—the belief that "it can't happen to me"—but many people continue to put themselves at risk of HIV/AIDS because their social and economic circumstances make it hard not to. Chapter 1 outlined the many ways in which poverty reduces people's ability to control their lives. If some homosexual men have modified their behaviour it is because as a group they have considerable advantages which others lack: a strong identity, relative wealth and autonomy, a supportive network and emerging political strength. The lesson to be learnt from this is that ensuring awareness of HIV/AIDS is not enough to generate behaviour change: other conditions also have to be met.

Conditions for Change

People will adopt safer sexual practices only if three conditions are met: they must have access to information; they must have access to condoms; and, most importantly, they must have the power to implement safer sexual practices.

Access to information

Information on HIV/AIDS and the means of preventing transmission needs to be culturally appropriate and widely available in the daily spoken language of the target audience. Where literacy levels are low, the information must be passed on orally or graphically, through such means as community groups, street theatre or one-to-one counselling. Education campaigns

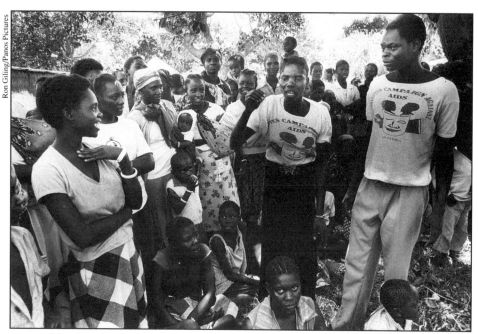

Ron Giling/Panos Pictures

Education through drama: a theatre group in Zambia takes information about HIV/AIDS from village to village.

have used puppet theatre in South Africa, folklore and religion in the Dominican Republic and animated clay figures in Brazil. Traditional dance has been a medium of education in Thailand, where many channels of communication are encouraged to present information on the disease, involving diverse elements of society—from the film industry to Buddhist monks.

Access to condoms

Condoms need to be easily available at no cost or at a price the individual can afford. Social marketing—the application of commercial sales and marketing skills to public health problems—can help recover some of the costs and improve access, and help dispel some of the negative connotations of condom use (see Box on p133).

Empowerment

An individual must have the power to change his or her behaviour if they wish to. This may mean challenging strongly held cultural notions about male and female sexuality, as well as addressing some of the economic inequalities which influence sexual decisionmaking.

According to Gary Slutkin, chief of Intervention Development and Support at the Global Programme on AIDS, three further conditions are necessary for the implementation of effective HIV/AIDS education.

Steps forward to gaining control

Empower is an organisation running drop-in centres and outreach programmes for women working in the sex industry of Bangkok and Chiang Mai, Thailand. With little or no control over their lives and working conditions, the women face many problems, of which HIV is only one. Empower therefore does not see AIDS as an issue which can be separated from the other issues it tackles on a daily basis.

The services offered by the drop-in centres have practical value but also enhance the women's self-confidence and ability to take some control over their lives, individually and collectively. There are classes in Thai, English, sewing, typing and drama. Throughout the year there is a choice of workshops in batik, photography, cooking and video-making. The women can also get advice on legal and health matters. Many contribute to the bi-monthly newsletter which unites the women in different areas. The centres also provide a focal point for women to meet and discuss family problems, share experiences, chat and relax together.

Learning English and Thai is important so that the women can insist on receiving the correct amount of money for their services and persuade customers to use condoms. In the workshops the women role-play such activities as getting rid of a customer who refuses to use a condom, questioning a doctor on the contraceptives he prescribes and presenting a proposal to a committee. Workshops are also opportunities to voice fears, angers and expectations. Some groups go out into the streets and bars to perform comic drama sketches which remind co-workers and customers of the need to use condoms.

Because many women are trapped into debt to the brothel owners—who lend money to their families—they are not free to leave the brothels and join in the centres' activities. So Empower staff take the newsletter and, in several places, the classes to the women. Sometimes English and Thai lessons are given—and watched by confused customers—in the glass-fronted areas where the girls have to display themselves. Through study the women acquire some self-esteem; some refuse to take customers during this hour and ask in indignation if the customers can't see that they are busy studying. They have also started to stop customers switching on the juke box while they study. Small steps, but steps forward: towards making the customer realise that these are women with desires and aspirations, studying like everyone else and worthy of respect; and towards demanding some time for themselves, questioning their lack of rights and being able to protect themselves by demanding the use of a condom.

Empower, *Thailand*

First, governments need to take policy decisions to initiate and allow HIV/AIDS prevention programmes. This must include guaranteeing freedom of speech to discuss all sexual and social issues underlying the epidemic.

Second, while the public needs to be informed via the mass media about the virus, this information must be complemented by peer education, in which trusted individuals from the same background as a target group encourage and enable them to change their behaviour. People with HIV/AIDS working as peer educators are particularly effective [9].

Third, care services need to be provided which are more than medical, and incorporate opportunities for counselling, thereby breaking down the stigma against HIV/AIDS and building up understanding in the patients' families and communities. Developed in this way, care services form an essential aspect of prevention [10].

Target Audiences

While everyone needs to be aware of the existence of HIV/AIDS and the means of protection, experience shows that interventions focused on clearly defined target groups have the best chance of success.

The mathematical models described in Chapter 2 back up this focused approach, since they showed how the rapid spread of HIV is enabled by frequent sexual partner change by a relatively small

Prevention through peer education

Hernan is 25, gay and comes from one of Lima's deprived neighbourhoods. "It's not easy to get a proper job with so much unemployment around," he says. "I have been a male prostitute for 10 years. I began partly for pleasure and partly for economic reasons."

Fortunately, Hernan knows how to protect himself from HIV, thanks to the intervention of Proyecto Germinal, an AIDS prevention project aimed at gay adolescents from marginalised urban areas. According to project coordinator Pepe Vargas: "In our society homosexuals are second-class citizens. They are rejected by all. As a result, they usually have very low self-esteem. We want to teach them to defend and enjoy their legitimate rights to life."

According to recent surveys, up to 83% of the Peruvian population are not in full-time formal employment. And in Peru's "macho" society, openly gay youths from poor backgrounds have few job opportunities beyond becoming cooks, hairdressers or *fletes* (prostitutes). When Hernan's first love relationship broke up, he began to go daily to meet new male partners at the Plaza San Martin (a meeting point for *fletes*) before and after school. It was there, waiting for clients, that he was recruited by Proyecto Germinal, for which he is now a workshop organiser.

Hernan knows that teenagers should be better informed about sex. "I had no advice at all from my parents about sex," he says. "I wanted to have sex—but I didn't know whether I wanted it with a girl or a boy. I was confused then. There was a boy in my neighbourhood to whom I was attracted. I had my first sexual experience with him."

Proyecto Germinal organisers help inform their members about HIV/AIDS prevention through discussions about safer sex and lifestyles which prevent infection. The group also helps those who are HIV-positive to cope with their situation and recognise their rights. Through stressing self-esteem, it hopes to empower youths who sell sex to demand that clients protect them by using condoms. In turn, members spread information on HIV/AIDS within the gay community.

Maritza Luque, *adapted from WorldAIDS, March 1992*

number of people. Reducing transmission in this group will have a far greater effect than reducing it among people with a low rate of partner change (see p26).

As well as sex workers, and people who frequently change sexual partners, key target groups include migrant workers, injecting drug users, young adults and adolescents. Peer education in prostitutes' groups has proved to be particularly successful. Women can also be reached through antenatal programmes, while men can be targeted through STD clinics.

Interventions focused on clearly defined target groups have the best chance of success

The workplace offers good opportunities for HIV/AIDS prevention programmes; in particular, they reach a large number of men. They also allow educators to target risk behaviour associated with working, such as the habit of drinking and having sex after work or when travelling away from home. Programmes specifically for truck-drivers and for other trades where men are away from their families for long periods have also had some success, although, depending on the sense of solidarity within the group, peer education may be more difficult and less effective than among women. Seven out of ten companies surveyed in Zambia either had an education programme or planned to introduce one [11]. The Brazilian Inter-disciplinary AIDS Association (ABIA) is an NGO which undertakes education programmes within commercial enterprises employing from 400 to 19,000 people (see overleaf) [12]. At each training course they ask companies to invite representatives of other businesses to be present. Similar programmes are under way in other countries (see Chapter 5).

Migrant workers can be approached through some of these same channels, as well as in bars, hostels and organisations where they congregate. Male bisexual behaviour is common in many parts of the world and programmes need to be designed for men who have sex with other men but who do not identify as gay.

Intervention programmes that have implicitly or explicitly taken into account the importance of carefully tailoring information, providing resources and addressing issues of powerlessness have achieved significant behaviour change within their target groups. Examples include women sex workers and their clients in Bulawayo in Zimbabwe [13] and Calabar in Nigeria [14], lorry drivers in Tanzania, military recruits in Rwanda [15], and sex workers in Mexico [16], Brazil [17] and Thailand [18]. But the total number involved is still only a small minority of the world's population who remain at risk of HIV/AIDS infection.

AIDS, business and videos

"If we are investing in training, then we have to be concerned with the health of our employees." The comment comes from Wilson Brumer, president of Companhia Vale do Rio Doce (CVRD) the fifth-ranking Brazilian company, with an annual turnover of $2.2 billion. Vale was established in 1942 and is an international company comprising mining and related industries. Its best known activity is the mining, transport and export of iron ore. It operates in nine states of Brazil, with headquarters in Rio de Janeiro.

The company's HIV/AIDS programme began in February 1991 with the assistance of ABIA. "The central idea", according to programme coordinator Oneida Enne, "is to enable our target audience to recognise the diverse aspects of the illness, act in a preventive manner, take on campaign tasks in the company itself and the communities it works in, and improve attitudes towards people with HIV/AIDS."

Not before time: if the number of reported AIDS cases in Brazil is near 30,000, the estimates of those infected are 20 times that figure. In this context, as Veronica Hughes of the education department of the AIDS Reference and Training Centre (São Paulo) points out: "It is natural that businesses with 5,000 or 10,000 employees have some cases [of HIV/AIDS]."

But it was not the number of cases in the company—so far no more than 10—which drew Vale's attention. What guided the company's approach was its traditional preoccupation with community support. After half a century exploiting non-renewable natural resources, the institution recognises its responsibility towards the ecological and socio-economic results of its activities. Public issues, such as epidemics, which affect the communities where Vale works are seen as institutional priorities.

CVRD's campaign consists of training "monitors" to familiarise small groups on HIV/AIDS. A programme is set up to inform the monitors and at the same time train them to disseminate the information further. The monitors are social assistants, health professionals, lawyers, engineers, supervisors, equipment operators, administrative agents and secretaries. Some are not employees, but members of the local communities.

To support these activities, Vale has published an education leaflet, printed T-shirts, key-rings and badges, and started a video library with films on AIDS. It has also organised events like "A Day for Life" and "A Week for Life"; the latter brought together 700 people in Rio de Janeiro. In company units with more employees, such as Vitória and São Luís, the campaign is more intensive, emphasising the involvement of health and social service personnel. In others, the stress is on awareness.

The company unit at Porto de Tubarão in Vitória, has produced the most innovative campaign. At Carnival in 1992, all the buses and cars entering the service terminal received leaflets and condoms, to the sound of a tune specially written for the campaign by an employee. The song is already on video, and is now circulating in other units.

Some 13,500 people are estimated to have been reached, both employees and people in the wider community, and 130 monitors have been trained. The annual cost of the campaign—including meetings, printed material and some travel expenses—is $28,000. Compared with the monthly cost of treating an employee with AIDS of at least $1,200 (not including indirect costs), prevention has an excellent cost to benefit ratio.

Enne says that feedback from the campaign has been encouraging: "The monitors have become sources of information for people both inside and outside the company. Requests for seminars, materials and help with campaigns are also increasing in other parts of the business. And there are changes in attitude. We had relations and colleagues of employees with AIDS participating in the 'Week for Life'. It has become easier to talk about the subject and in some cases the climate of fear has given way to solidarity. Also the number of people requesting HIV tests has risen. And in two places in the heart of the country Vale employees have joined community committees to fight AIDS."

The biggest challenge to this type of continuing campaign is creativity. Tackling the topic can wake up people's attention; the danger is making the issue banal through repetition.

Milton Quintino, *coordinator of Religious Support Against AIDS, Rio de Janeiro*

Today's children: tomorrow's adults

In almost every country a significant proportion of the population that contracts HIV does so in their teens. Whether their sexual activity begins early or late, within or outside marriage, adolescents need to be made aware of the nature of HIV/AIDS and the means to avoid it, before they become sexually active. Shyamala Nataraj, coordinator of the South India AIDS Action Programme, points out the dangers in India, where general awareness about HIV prevention is low amongst adolescents and where pre-marital sex and the sharing of needles for intravenous drug use are both on the increase. "Early education on sexuality, STDs and the ability to make responsible choices are therefore vital. In major cities, school and college authorities are now approaching AIDS workers to run awareness programmes for their students. Interest levels are high and students ask questions on sexual behaviour and risks that are obviously important to them. One student said: 'We cannot talk about our sexual feelings, or fears, with anybody. We wish we could.' Several groups are now focusing on educating adolescents in schools and colleges. However, it is doubtful if a fully fledged campaign that promotes condom use and makes them available will be launched. That will surely face much opposition. Yet until that is done the Indian adolescent will continue to be vulnerable to HIV and other STDs [19]."

Some argue that sex education encourages sexual activity and experimentation and therefore might lead to more, not less, transmission of HIV. However, Michael Merson, director of WHO's Global Programme on AIDS, points out: "Research has shown that, contrary to popular belief, children who receive sex education do not become sexually active earlier than others. Quite the opposite: such youngsters delay their sexual experimentation, and when they do engage in intercourse, they are more likely to take the right precautions, including contraception [20]."

Many of the people who contract HIV do so in their teens; HIV awareness helps this particularly vulnerable group to protect themselves. This popular magazine has introduced the subject to schools in Kenya.

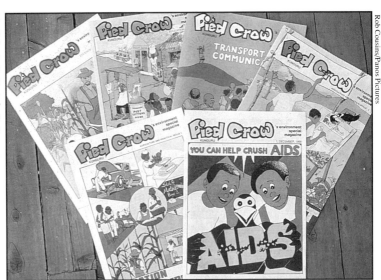

One of the best known programmes has been the anti-AIDS clubs set up by children throughout Zambia, where all members agree to abstain from sexual intercourse before marriage. The clubs not only spread information about HIV/AIDS among children and foster greater awareness of the consequences, but also, according to Susan Foster of the ADZAM study, have a wider influence, making adults more willing to change their behaviour. Evidence is also emerging from some areas where the epidemic has been widespread, that high school children are less likely to engage in sexual intercourse [21]. One novel idea has been to suggest that a pass mark in nationwide exams be dependent on knowledge of HIV/AIDS prevention [22].

Counselling and Care

Behaviour change may also result from targeted programmes that have other primary objectives, such as those designed to care for and counsel those who are HIV-positive or who have developed AIDS. These services usually draw in the patients' partners, families and friends and have proved to have considerable prevention potential [23].

The drawback of counselling is that it is labour-intensive. Laurie Liskin of Johns Hopkins University in the USA points out: "While new approaches are widening the reach of counselling services, it is clear that counselling is not a simple or quick route to behaviour change. In [one Zairean] study, for example, discordant couples [where one partner is HIV-positive and the other is HIV-negative] needed repeated counselling visits both at

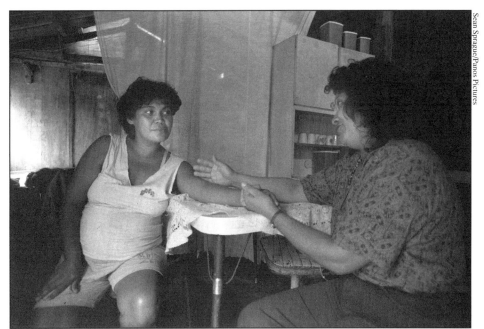

A counsellor visits a pregnant woman who is HIV-positive in São Paulo, Brazil. Caring for people in the community has proved an effective way of spreading information about the disease and encouraging prevention.

home and in the clinic to help them cope with the stress of an HIV-positive diagnosis and to maintain safe sexual practices." In Mexico at least three months of weekly group therapy sessions were needed to increase condom use among infected homosexual men who remained sexually active [24].

Michael Merson states: "Care for infected people is indispensable—to keep their dignity intact and their hope alive, to encourage their families to stand by them and not reject them, and hence to avoid social disintegration [25]." Isolating patients fuels stigma; the more the community knows about AIDS, the more chance there is to combat its spread. The difficulty is proving this statistically. Sue Lucas, of the UK NGO AIDS Consortium for the Third World, points out that "care is often poorly funded because many donors want statistical proof that care leads to prevention. For example, USAID is one major donor that [does not] fund care programmes [26]."

Horizontal and vertical programmes

Development agencies describe programmes focusing exclusively on HIV/AIDS awareness and prevention as "vertical" and programmes which integrate this into other activities as "horizontal". Some development workers feel that HIV/AIDS interventions "reinvent the wheel" by creating new mechanisms —NGOs, offices, administrative facilities—where they already

Successful interventions recognise the social factors that allow the virus to spread

exist to deal with other health or development issues. Experience suggests, however, that in countries where HIV/AIDS has recently appeared or there is little public knowledge of the disease and its means of transmission, vertical programmes are the only effective means of raising awareness. From Gay Men's Health Crisis in New York to Pink Triangle in Malaysia and the Brazilian Inter-disciplinary AIDS Association (ABIA), the first response to the epidemic has frequently come from NGOs set up specifically to address the issue.

In countries where the epidemic is endemic and its threat widely recognised, integrated programmes are more appropriate. An institution offering one service, such as family planning advice, primary health care or STD treatment, is often well-placed to expand its activities to include HIV/AIDS.

Sexual Health

Many see strengthening STD control programmes as a priority, both because the spread of HIV is directly assisted by other untreated STDs and in order to provide a framework for counselling and education about HIV/AIDS, and condom distribution. This will often require active government intervention.

Mike Bailey, a specialist on HIV/AIDS and development who has worked with UNDP, suggests that in many countries ministries of health pay little attention to STD prevention since it is easier to prescribe treatment for a disease than to counsel for its prevention [27]—and in the past even treatment for STDs has often been unavailable or unaffordable. However, improving STD programmes could be seen as a "no-risk strategy" in that whatever course the HIV epidemic takes, there are definite benefits in reducing the high and rising rates of STDs, which are associated with infertility, still-births and general health complications. A nationwide STD programme in Zambia, with an annual budget of $700,000 has seen the number of reported STDs fall dramatically since 1988, and the incidence of genital ulcers has been halved [28].

However, integrating HIV/AIDS prevention into other activities is not merely a case of offering information. Successful interventions are those which recognise and respond to the social and psychological factors that allow the virus to spread. A family planning clinic that does no more than offer information on HIV on the same basis as offering information on different forms of contraception, may have little impact on the epidemic.

Condoms: barriers to acceptance

Condoms provide a physical barrier that significantly reduces transmission of HIV and other STDs. Under test conditions condoms have a high rate of reliability, but poor manufacture, deterioration in storage and conditions in actual use may severely reduce that reliability.

A number of factors limit widespread condom use, particularly in the developing world. These include problems of distribution and cost: the typical price of a condom, 20-50 US cents, makes it a luxury for those whose income may be no more than $20 a month. In addition, there are often strong sociological, psychological and physical factors which discourage individuals from using condoms. To ensure successful condom use, men and women must:

* take the decision to use them;
* know how to use them;
* have them easily available;
* be able to persuade a potentially reluctant partner to use them;
* be able to refuse intercourse with those who decline to use them;
* be able to dispose of used condoms.

Condom distribution has risen significantly in many parts of the world in recent years. Although distribution of free condoms is often erratic, social marketing is proving successful in a number of countries, raising the sale of condoms from 100,000 a year in 1987 to 18 million a year in 1991 in Zaire [50]. A number of studies at the Dakar conference on AIDS in Africa, in December 1991, reported success in raising the distribution of condoms in different countries [51].

However, strong opposition to use of condoms remains. Married women in some countries have protested against their husbands receiving condoms on the grounds that it encourages them to have extra-marital affairs. "Many people associate condoms with prostitution and illicit sex," according to Samson Kisekka, vice-president of Uganda. "Therefore married couples and men who fear being branded as promiscuous do not use them [52]."

Elsewhere, for example in India, condom use may have the opposite association—men who use them within marriage for contraceptive purposes do not use them with prostitutes. In many cases condoms are rejected because of perceptions that they reduce pleasure. Where one person accepts use of a condom, their partner may not—and a woman's power to insist on safe sex may be limited. It may mean risking the loss of the emotional or financial support of her partner. The desire to have children is another common reason for not using condoms.

For these and other reasons, some prevention programmes, particularly those sponsored by religious organisations, argue that condoms are not the answer to HIV/AIDS.

Even where condoms are available and acceptable, practical problems can arise. In parts of India there are complaints that the wrong type of condom (non-lubricated) is distributed through the primary health care system [53]. A report on condom use in rural Kenya found that lack of access to lighting and water—to check the condoms for possible tears and to wash hands after use—were compounded by problems of disposal [54].

One of the problems of family planning programmes is that they tend to focus on women, with the result that men have not been helpful to their female partners in managing contraceptive problems. Given that the one available effective means of preventing transmission of HIV and other STDs—condoms —requires full participation of the male partner, more attention must be given to the sexual and reproductive needs of men [29]. That is why some experts call for a movement towards sexual health programmes, which would integrate all the different aspects of sexual health such as family planning, the prevention of STDs and HIV/AIDS, infertility and so on.

Measuring results

The clearest evidence of behaviour change is proven long-term reduction in the rate of new HIV infections in a target group. However, apart from gay men in the industrialised world, this is relatively rare. A second measurement, particularly where HIV infection rates are low, is a fall in the rate of new infections of other sexually transmitted diseases. Another barometer is the extent to which sales or distribution of condoms have increased, as has been seen in a growing number of countries and in certain population groups.

In addition to such measurable behaviour change, evidence is emerging that in many parts of Africa people are modifying their sex lives. A study in Kampala, Uganda, sees an increase in monogamy and a reduction in HIV rates of infection among young adults, but it is not yet possible to say whether this is a definite trend [30].

Sue Lucas, of the UK NGO AIDS Consortium for the Third World, has been getting strong anecdotal evidence from African NGOs that there are fewer people visiting bars, less ritual cleansing (the practice whereby a man has sexual intercourse with his brother's widow) and more people coming forward to be trained as educators, all of which indicate people are responding positively to the epidemic.

Lucas argues that such changes are not widely reported or recognised because they are the result of interventions undertaken by local community-based organisations with little experience of presenting information in the style traditionally demanded by donors. This difficulty of communication between funders and funded can mean that the former are left uncertain as to which approaches have the most impact and therefore how best to allocate resources [31].

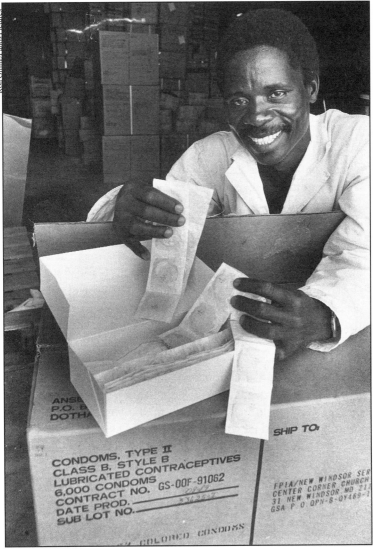

Condom distribution is the simple aspect of intervention programmes, but to be effective it must be accompanied by education campaigns which address the various objections to condom use.

The Cost of Interventions

Interventions not only save illness and lives, they make economic sense. Costs may appear high, but they are significantly lower than the costs of sickness and death resulting from HIV/AIDS.

Condom distribution is the simplest aspect of intervention programmes. It has been estimated that to provide a couple with two condoms per week costs an average of $6.45 per year [32]. If 50% of a country's population is sexually active and uses condoms at this rate, annual expenditure on condoms will come to $1.65 per capita. These figures compare with the typical $5 per

Interventions   capita currently spent on all health care in some of the countries
make   worst-affected by the epidemic.
economic   No condom distribution will be effective without extensive
sense   education programmes to ensure that the condoms are actually
used. The US agency AIDSTECH is assisting the Commercial
Farmers Union (CFU) of Zimbabwe in an education programme
which includes free condom distribution. According to Peter
Fraser-Mackenzie of the CFU, the programme costs farmers
roughly Z$10 (US$2) a year per employee, with condoms the
most expensive element [33]. In the Mutorashanga area, where
the scheme has been operating for some time, condoms are widely
available and the incidence of STDs reported at the local clinic
has declined [34].

The US agency Family Health International (FHI) has
calculated the average cost of education and condom distribution
programmes in parts of Latin America and the Caribbean as $6.70
per commercial sex worker per month. The cost of preventing
one primary infection (infection in the target group), is calculated
as between $312 and $9,069 (average $3,041). If between two
and six secondary infections (infections in sexual partners of the
target group) were prevented for every primary infection
prevented, cost per infection prevented drops to $45-$3,023 [35].

Taking these figures one step further, FHI analysed the
potential savings of a programme in comparison to the cost of
treating an individual with HIV/AIDS. Assuming a low figure of
$3,300 as treatment costs in Latin America and the Caribbean,
the conclusion was that the direct benefits of preventing future
treatment costs would be between 3.5 and 7.5 times greater
(depending on the number of secondary infections prevented)
than the cost of the intervention [36].

Preliminary results from an FHI study in Zimbabwe, where
both prevention costs and treatment are much lower, indicate that
the cost per primary infection averted is $11, while the benefits
were 36 times greater than the costs of intervention [37]. These
figures apply to treatment only. If the medical and lost labour
costs in Central Africa are taken, as in World Bank studies, as a
theoretical average of $3,000 per capita [38], 99% of this figure
would be saved. Similar prevention costs, of $8 to $12 per case
averted, were calculated in Kenya [39].

Even assuming far greater prevention costs, including the costs
of blood screening, administration etc, interventions still provide
significant cost-benefit. A 1987 model of HIV/AIDS activities in
Burundi, which included treatment and preventing infection

through blood transfusion, infected needles and sexual transmission (through nationwide rather than targeted intervention), estimated overall costs as between $413,000 and $630,000 per 100,000 people, depending on the rate of infection. The cost of HIV prevention would be between $164 and $868 per case averted [40].

Information is a prerequisite but not a guarantee of change

The Thai study, on the basis of the $100 million spent in 1991-92, suggests that interventions may result in 3.5 million fewer people becoming infected and $5.1 billion being saved. Even if the annual AIDS prevention budget were to triple, the cost of prevention would yield a 17 times return on that investment [41].

Despite the obvious savings generated by successful interventions, actual spending is far lower than required. WHO's figure of $0.46 per person per year spent on all HIV/AIDS-related activities is matched by the Global AIDS Policy Coalition's figure of $169 million as the average annual donation by governments and NGOs in the North to the developing world for HIV/AIDS activities between 1987 and 1991 [42]. This is a fraction—0.3%—of the Official Development Assistance (ODA) for developing countries in 1990. After reaching a peak of $255 million in 1990, international funding of the WHO-sponsored global AIDS strategy fell to $237 million in 1991 [43], and there is no sign of this trend being reversed.

Political will

There is no easy solution to the problem of reducing HIV transmission. Information is a prerequisite but not a guarantee of change. Programmes cannot be implemented in isolation from the circumstances of people's lives, and a wide-ranging approach, involving different sectors of the community, is necessary.

Roy Anderson's team at Imperial College, London, calls for priority to be given to scientific assessment of different intervention strategies, such as education, condom distribution or STD treatment, and for studies of behaviour both before and after a given intervention: "In addition to measuring success via changes in rates of infection, emphasis should be placed on assessing precisely who changes behaviour and why, and how behavioural changes influence networks of sexual contacts within populations [44]." WHO is coordinating a number of such studies, but results are not yet available.

While individuals need to have the information, the will and above all the power to protect themselves, political will is another essential element—and one which in most countries has been present more in speeches than in practice. As one paper pointed

Actions have to be taken on evidence of potential rather than actual spread

out: "The reluctance of politicians to launch health education campaigns that talk openly about sex, condom use and reduction of promiscuity is universal [45]." Health ministries obviously play a key role in raising public awareness, but health ministers generally have less influence in governments than their colleagues in finance, home or foreign affairs. And because of the submerged nature of the disease in many countries, actions have to be taken on evidence of potential rather than actual spread. Yet it is at this point, before the virus has taken hold, that the implementation of interventions is most cost-effective. It may be that it is only when the prime minister or president becomes convinced of the threat of AIDS—as in Thailand and Uganda—that governments become fully involved. Finally, given that HIV/AIDS is increasingly a disease of disadvantage, there needs to be the political will to tackle inequalities and improve the social and economic circumstances of the world's poor.

CHAPTER 9

A development issue

In the 1980s, the international response to the appearance of HIV/AIDS was to treat the epidemic as an emergency issue. Hundreds of millions of dollars were spent in supporting a wide range of interventions. In the 1990s, it is clear the epidemic has become endemic—a phenomenon that will persist in many communities for many years to come.

In the North the severity of the epidemic varies, but it is a problem that can be contained well within each country's resources. The picture in the developing world is very different. Some countries are already in danger of being overwhelmed by the epidemic; others—not all of which have recognised or acknowledged the threat—have many people HIV-positive but relatively few diagnosed with AIDS. The majority of developing countries, including those worst affected, have few financial and technical resources with which to limit the spread and the impact of the disease. Most are struggling to improve the quality of life for their people at all levels: to reduce poverty and increase equity, to raise levels of education, health and nutrition. All these aspects of development impinge upon the spread of HIV/AIDS: any improvement in the social and economic conditions of poorer people's lives reduces their vulnerability to the disease.

The Role of Development

"Development" means different things to different people and communities. Some stress economic growth, others emphasise social development, preferring to focus on distribution rather than generation of income. Most, however, would now agree that it includes both social and economic factors. The first *Human Development Report,* published in 1990 by the United Nations Development Programme, was a recognition that measuring development by economic indicators alone conceals more than it reveals. It now publishes annually the Human Development Index, which takes account of more human factors such as life expectancy, health, and educational attainment, as well as GNP.

HIV/AIDS is both a symptom and increasingly a cause of under-development It defines development as enlarging the range of people's choices—for example, increasing their opportunities for education, health care, income, employment, and to live in a safe physical environment. Development may be achieved through the actions of individuals, community-based organisations, governments and international organisations, but without the participation of the people it seeks to benefit, the chances of lasting effectiveness are slim.

The extent to which development strategies of the last few decades have been successful is a matter of widespread debate: some communities and countries in the developing world, mostly in Asia, have achieved significant improvements in living standards; others, mostly in Africa, have seen increasing rates of poverty, malnutrition and disease. Meanwhile, the process of development continues to be hampered by a global economy that encourages a flow of wealth from poor nations to rich nations, and the exploitation of resources at an unsustainable rate.

Worldwide, 0.3% of annual financial aid from industrialised countries to developing countries is spent on HIV/AIDS [1]. Clearly, out of the many sectors and activities competing for attention and funding, the epidemic has been for many agencies a relatively low priority. Nonetheless, the fact that HIV/AIDS is both a symptom and increasingly a cause of underdevelopment is a strong argument for continuing and indeed raising the level of funding of HIV/AIDS prevention and care. Wealth and health are two sides of the same coin; if one is threatened, so is the other. The rapid spread of HIV/AIDS can be partly attributed to the failure of development; and it will increasingly contribute to that failure. An effective response to the epidemic can therefore be seen as a development priority.

Many different agencies are involved in development. They include small community-based organisations, such as market traders' and tenants' associations; non-government organisations (NGOs) of all sizes and complexion; religious organisations; the business community; women's groups; trade unions; government ministries; donor organisations; and United Nations agencies. Money and experience flows through this complicated web, sometimes effectively, sometimes dissipated through mismanagement, bureaucracy or corruption. Development is not an exact science: different theories have been promoted and then lost favour, and there have been plenty of misjudgements and misunderstandings, many rooted in the tendency of donors to impose their ideas of development on recipients.

This tendency has increasingly been acknowledged as one of the reasons why the millions of dollars poured into aid since the 1960s have not had greater effect. A huge and complicated aid industry has grown up to deliver financial and technical resources, but at the heart of development are the actions of individuals and communities, whose own views, values and experiences have often been swamped or ignored by the machinery of aid. Without their determination, resourcefulness, energy and commitment, development cannot take place. The aid network can play an important role in development, but it is not the central part.

The most vigorous response to the epidemic has come from individuals and communities

In HIV/AIDS, as in other aspects of development, the most vigorous response to the epidemic has come from individuals and communities, but their efforts will be far less fruitful if they do not have wider support. Indeed, as this dossier points out, the potential cost of HIV/AIDS is so enormous that external assistance is vital. The next section looks at some of the organisations responsible for delivering this assistance.

Multilaterals and bilaterals

Bilateral aid is dispersed on a country-to-country basis, through national agencies such as the UK Overseas Development Administration (ODA), the US Agency for International Development (USAID) and the Danish International Development Agency (DANIDA).

Bilateral aid has been a significant source of funds for HIV/AIDS interventions in the developing world. Agencies have different policies and priorities in terms of projects and partners. USAID, for example, will not fund treatment programmes and works directly with a narrow range of institutions; the Canadian International Development Agency (CIDA) and the Norwegian Agency for International Development (NORAD) frequently work directly with small NGOs; the Netherlands Foreign Ministry places a strong emphasis on human rights in its funding.

Multilateral agencies are intergovernmental organisations, to which individual countries contribute funds. Examples are the World Health Organization (WHO), Food and Agriculture Organization (FAO) and other specialised UN agencies. The first UN agency to respond to the epidemic was WHO, which established the Special Programme on AIDS, later renamed the Global Programme on AIDS (GPA), in 1986. The following year the United Nations passed a resolution which called on the Secretary-General, in conjunction with WHO, to ensure a coordinated response by the UN system to the pandemic. By the

UNDP strategy

The United Nations Development Programme (UNDP) has drawn up a strategy for dealing with HIV/AIDS in the 1990s. Parts of that strategy are outlined here.

UNDP will:

- increase awareness of the development implications of the epidemic;
- strengthen and expand the capacity of communities to respond to the epidemic;
- promote and assist prevention, care, support and treatment programmes for women;
- assist governments to develop effective multisectoral HIV/AIDS strategies and to minimise the devastating consequences of widespread infection.

UNDP's long-term goals are to:

- prevent further transmission of HIV, in particular through behaviour change;
- strengthen the coping capacities and strategies of affected individuals, families, communities, business and governments;
- develop multidisciplinary and multisectoral approaches to minimise the adverse social and economic consequences of the epidemic.

UNDP's priorities include:

- advocacy—increasing awareness of the epidemic, the implications for economic and social development and the need for urgent, effective action;
- national policy development—assisting governments to develop HIV/AIDS-related policies;
- women—addressing women's needs for prevention, care, support and access to treatment.

The policy issues surrounding this epidemic are complex and will change as the pattern and impact of the epidemic evolves. Policies must remain responsive to this change.

- An integrated and comprehensive approach must be based on an understanding of the way HIV/AIDS affects personal, social and economic development.
- The coping strategies of communities must be central to the national response; community-based organisations will be instrumental in ensuring human survival, human rights and human development.
- Policies relating to HIV/AIDS must encompass and be accepted by all sectors in society. Those affected by the epidemic should be involved in the policy dialogue.
- A proper balance must be found among programmes for prevention, social support, research and development.
- In order to be successful, programmes must take into account and explore each culture's ability to evolve and change in response to the challenge of the epidemic.
- The power imbalances which create women's subordination must change if women are to be able to protect themselves from HIV infection and its consequences.
- Each individual has the responsibility to protect himself or herself from HIV/AIDS and to minimise further spread of the epidemic.
- The means of reducing the risk of HIV transmission must be affordable by and accessible to everyone.
- The cooperation and trust of people at risk of infection must be established and maintained.
- The rights of people with HIV/AIDS must be respected and those affected must remain an integral part of the community.

Source: UNDP DP/1991/57

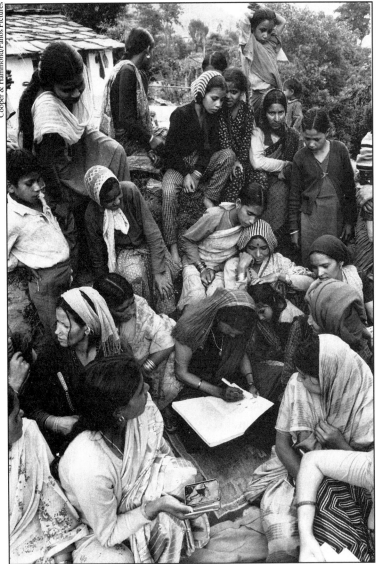

A women's savings group in North India, meeting to discuss and find their own solutions to local problems.

end of the 1980s, almost all UN agencies had discussed the issue and adopted resolutions appropriate to their field.

GPA has been the most active and interventionist of WHO's programmes, sponsoring the establishment of National AIDS Control Programmes in over 160 countries, and directly supporting NGOs throughout the developing world. Its annual budget reached $100 million in 1990, but fell back to $87 million in 1991 [2], partly as a result of donor governments, who provide the bulk of the income, diverting funds directly to HIV/AIDS programmes in specific countries.

Perhaps inevitably for a programme that grew so quickly, GPA has been criticised on a number of grounds; these include lack of sensitivity to specific country needs, and concentration on prevention at the expense of care [3]. Its stated priorities for the 1990s—vaccine development, clinical research and drug development, improvement in diagnostics and epidemiological research—have also been criticised, on the grounds of not placing enough emphasis on care or ensuring availability of existing drugs in the developing world. However, its coordinating role, its access to governments worldwide and the resources it commands, ensure that it has played and will continue to play a pivotal role in responding to the pandemic.

While GPA focuses on medical aspects of HIV/AIDS, the approach of the United Nations Development Programme (UNDP) has been to increase awareness of the development implications of the pandemic and strengthen response to the problems that it causes. UNDP, considered to be at the centre of the UN's development efforts, has set out a series of principles to guide policy development (see p142), brought together experts on the issue and supported a range of interventions in a number of countries.

Other multilateral agencies which have addressed the issue include the International Labour Organization, UNICEF and FAO, which has sponsored research into the impact of the epidemic on agriculture (see Chapter 6). The World Bank funds studies of the economic implications of HIV/AIDS, a number of which have been reported in this dossier. Most concentrate on sub-Saharan Africa and include detailed reports jointly prepared with the governments of Tanzania and Uganda.

Government response
The response of individual governments within developing countries to the epidemic has generally been coordinated by National AIDS Control Programmes (NACPs) set up at the instigation and with the cooperation of WHO. In the 1980s, the primary role of NACPs was to oversee one-year plans that estimated the extent of the epidemic and where possible and appropriate, to take immediate action in areas such as blood screening. In the mid-1990s, NACPs are, at least theoretically, implementing three- to five-year plans which include interventions intended to bring about behaviour change. The programmes and budgets of these plans are devised in cooperation with WHO, and money is either allocated from current government funds or sought from donors.

The efficiency and impact of NACPs varies from country to country. Although many plans are being implemented successfully, others suffer from poor management and insufficient funding. NGOs frequently complain that their programmes are held up while they wait for government approval or for overseas funding if this has to go through government channels. A mid-term review of one country's five-year plan mentioned a lack of coordination between ministries and departments and that bureaucratic procedures were hindering the availability of funds. In addition, there was no national STD control programme, and inadequate facilities at the primary teaching hospital had precluded the establishment of a special HIV/AIDS clinic [4]. A further general criticism of government response is that, with very few exceptions, the medical aspects of the epidemic are overemphasised at the expense of the social and economic dimensions.

In almost every country the first response has come from NGOs rather than government

NGOs

An enormous variety of NGOs is active in development. Some are operational, others are purely campaigning and lobbying organisations, others concentrate on research or education. They range from Northern-based agencies with million dollar budgets, such as the Ford Foundation and Oxfam, to small community-based organisations trying to respond to local needs with few resources beyond their members' time and commitment.

In almost every country the first response to HIV/AIDS has come from NGOs rather than government. There are hundreds of such organisations, covering a range of different concerns. Examples include TASO (The AIDS Support Organisation) in Uganda, which provides care and support for people with HIV/AIDS; Empower, which works with women prostitutes in Thailand; Dost, which runs a magazine and resource centre for gay men in India; and CEPSS, which runs a series of prevention programmes in the far south of Chile. The strength of community-based NGOs—in all areas of development—is that they usually have far greater understanding of the problems to be tackled and are more likely to have the confidence of the population concerned. This is particularly important for HIV/AIDS programmes, as trust is an essential first step to behaviour change. Many of the HIV/AIDS NGOs also see human rights and tackling the inequalities that allow the virus to spread as integral to their work.

Many other types of organisation are active in HIV/AIDS prevention. Churches and other religious groups have run

NGO policy in the 1990s

ACORD is an international consortium of non-government agencies implementing long-term development programmes in Africa. Its approach is to integrate its programmes into existing village structures rather than to set up new projects. In East Africa, ACORD works in Rwanda, Tanzania and Uganda. In this region, concludes a report by the NGO, it has become clear that "the current scale of the epidemic is such that one can no longer talk of 'vulnerable groups' or 'vulnerable areas': the entire population is affected, either directly or indirectly [12]." At the request of its programme staff, who are all nationals of the countries concerned, ACORD is devising a policy to respond to HIV/AIDS, both within the context of current programmes and as the basis of new initiatives.

ACORD programmes have several characteristics which should assist their work in HIV/AIDS. They have close village-level contacts with the rural population; experience suggests close and continous contact with the concerned communities is essential for HIV/AIDS work. It also has a "holistic" approach, as opposed to a sector by sector focus. ACORD sees the integration of HIV/AIDS activities into other areas of work as an overriding consideration. The approach is not to think of an "AIDS programme", but rather of a programme which answers the development needs of the community in the context of the HIV/AIDS epidemic. Any activity that improves people's environment and well-being, such as nutritional status, sanitation programmes etc, will be a step forward in combating the epidemic and its impact.

ACORD sees its role not as providing condoms, counselling or medical assistance, but as encouraging the emergence of local coping mechanisms, and supporting existing structures. It will actively bring individuals and communities together to discuss and exchange experiences in HIV/AIDS and support programmes by providing information, experience and research coordination. It believes that responses to the epidemic are more likely to be successful if they involve not just the individual, but the family and society, and if they are integrated within all other forms of interventions. The empowerment of women is essential.

ACORD's experience in Uganda highlighted several problems which have to be overcome in integrating and/or establishing HIV/AIDS programmes. These include difficulties in convincing colleagues who believe either that the epidemic is out of control, or is not a development issue; a heavy work-load which does not allow workers to take on HIV/AIDS; lack of funds; difficulty in collaborating with other institutions working in HIV/AIDS; too few teaching aids or none available in the local language; and an inability to respond to individual needs.

ACORD's response in Uganda has been to:

• intensify and broaden education campaigns, particularly to include such topics as legal awareness for women, sex education by parents, strengthening women's ability to say "no", and the need for community solidarity towards people with HIV/AIDS, guardians and orphans;

• support community-based mechanisms by such means as fostering the emergence of guardians' groups, providing seed money for income-generating activities, and training individuals as HIV/AIDS counsellors;

• sponsor research into labour-saving technologies, alternative income-generating activities for women, and integrating herbalists and other practitioners of traditional medicine into HIV/AIDS information and education activities.

These activities will be undertaken by reinforcing the capacity of existing community structures, such as rural development committees and village health committees. Wherever possible, people with AIDS will be encouraged to involve themselves in the programme.

The economic impact of the epidemic requires a broad response, going beyond the education and care activities just described. ACORD proposes new programmes such as:

- setting up locally-managed "solidarity shops" selling commodities produced through income-generating schemes linked to people affected by HIV/AIDS;
- broadening the range of income-generating opportunities for people with HIV/AIDS;
- launching credit schemes designed for people with HIV/AIDS, in collaboration with other NGOs involved in credit provision.

ACORD will also support research into the following:

- sexual behaviour;
- traditional medicine and the role practitioners could play in containing the epidemic;
- agricultural production techniques to replace labour-intensive practices which cannot be undertaken by people with HIV/AIDS.

In common with most NGOs, a key goal of ACORD is that programmes should aim to sustain themselves and not be dependent on outside assistance. However, some kinds of sustainability may not be possible with HIV/AIDS; for example, financial assistance given to people who are terminally ill is unlikely to be recovered. Of greater importance, ACORD believes, is the sustainability of the mechanisms and institutions set up. Ultimately, however, although ACORD may provide the impetus, local structures will have to develop their own mechanisms to ensure a degree of financial and institutional sustainability, however precarious that may be.

hospitals and clinics in the developing world for many years; commercial enterprises provide education for their employees, as seen in Chapter 5, and support campaigns aimed at a broader public; and academic institutions increase understanding of the pandemic through research. The media also have a role to play in increasing awareness, although in many countries sensationalist and inaccurate reporting has done more harm than good.

Barriers to Action

A WHO/UNDP statement points out: "Countries engaged in AIDS prevention and control have expressed concern about uncoordinated, ill-timed or inappropriate offers of external assistance to combat AIDS. Similarly, in order to ensure relevant, effective and efficient action, donor agencies have insisted on well coordinated activities in countries as a prerequisite for their support [5]."

Many of the countries and communities confronted by the epidemic are strong in human resources, but lack money and expertise. The costs of intervention in developing countries may

Donors are sometimes viewed as too restrictive in their conditions

be low in comparison with those in the industrialised world, but without external assistance they are often beyond the means of those who most need to undertake them. However, effective assistance is often hampered by barriers that arise between the three major players in HIV prevention: Northern/multilateral donors, Southern governments and Southern NGOs. These barriers include the following:

- Bureaucratic delays: usually caused by the demands of administration, most commonly from Northern donors and Southern governments. Simplifying accounting procedures would help, so that organisations would not have to support a full-time administration structure. Fully trained accountants are often few and far between.

- Different perceptions and priorities: donors and recipients may not agree how funds are best spent. This may stem from different priorities and also experiences; it may be hard to find a balance between a donor's experience of HIV/AIDS programmes at a global level and a community's understanding of local needs and values.

- Lack of experience: the enthusiasm of newly formed community-based organisations may not be matched by the necessary management skills.

- Denial: the refusal to acknowledge that HIV/AIDS exists in a community or is a problem can seriously delay prevention efforts. Governments may discourage open discussion of sexual behaviour, drug use or other factors behind the spread of HIV.

- Political considerations: NGOs may feel that government response is slow and subject more to political considerations than to the pressures of the epidemic. In some countries, NGOs have been extremely critical of their government's response, while some of those working in NACPs and ministries of health are suspicious of individuals and institutions who work outside the official network.

Some difficulties can be minimised, but solutions are not always easy. For example, to overcome delays caused by bureaucracy or lack of experience, donors may be willing to simplify accounting and reporting procedures but be unable to do so because they themselves are subject to stringent scrutiny.

Tensions can be eased if major donors and NGOs are represented on the committees that run National AIDS Control Programmes. NACPs with such a base are more likely to represent the broader needs of the community and to resolve

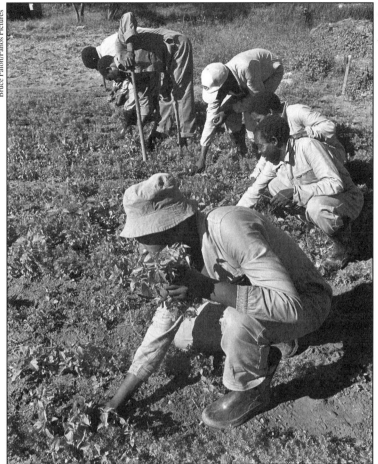

Bruce Paton/Panos Pictures

Agricultural training programmes, like this one under way in Zimbabwe, may need increasingly to take account of the needs of farmers losing labour and income because of HIV/AIDS.

conflicts before they arise. Many national AIDS committees, however, are composed primarily of medical personnel, and even those which are more broadly based seldom have representatives of the worst-affected communities or members who are publicly known to be HIV-positive.

Conflict between governments and NGOs can be reduced by greater recognition that each has different priorities and areas of expertise. According to Sue Lucas of the UK NGO AIDS Consortium for the Third World: "There's a whole area of debate about what is being expected of NGOs. It is not the role of NGOs to research and predict the impact of the epidemic. They should not be doing nationwide strategic planning. That is the task of governments. NGOs know what they should be doing but may not be articulating it very well. NGOs have local and specific expertise which should be built into national plans." Lucas argues that NGOs cannot and should not take on the role of providing

HIV/AIDS will not be contained as long as it is regarded as a health issue

national infrastructure, although in some countries up to 50% of hospital beds are provided by NGOs [6].

Mazuwa Banda of the Churches Medical Association has described how in Zambia there has evolved a "more or less workable arrangement whereby the government coordinates AIDS activities but does not necessarily control them" and does not insist on all money and expertise being channelled through it. The government considers any new initiatives and might step in if activities do not fall within the agreed broad framework. The high number of NGOs involved in Zambia means communication between each other and with the government can break down, so in 1989 the NGOs formed a coordinating structure: the National NGO Network on AIDS. This publishes a directory identifying the organisations and their work, to encourage the best use of available resources and avoid duplication. By 1992 there were well over 30 registered NGOs.

While cooperation and communication in Zambia has been good, says Banda, there is room for improvement. There has been an effort to get other ministries involved and take up AIDS components in their work; so far the ministries of education and of labour have responded. And while there is generally little friction between the government and donors, the latter sometimes feel the capacity to utilise funds is lacking and so are reluctant to donate. They also feel organisations are sometimes slow in meeting the demands of accountability. On the other hand, donors are sometimes viewed as being too restrictive in their conditions, or inflexible in their views. For example, they may earmark funds for a mass-media campaign, when the government and national NGOs perceive much greater needs in other areas. Sometimes this means one sector or organisation may receive a lot of money because donors are sympathetic to its methods or viewpoint. International NGO donors such as Oxfam are generally viewed as more flexible and comprehensive in their approach.

One difficulty, argues Banda, is that most donors do not recognise that HIV/AIDS is only one part of a problem and that in order to combat it strong infrastructure is needed. Less support is given to STD control, for example, because donors feel it is not their responsibility to fund care and treatment programmes. Similarly, it is much more difficult to get funds to deal with TB than HIV/AIDS, but "once TB gets out of hand there will be fewer resources on AIDS as people fire-fight TB and abandon AIDS programmes". By adopting a more comprehensive approach, it would be possible to minimise such conflicts [7].

"An Unprecedented Challenge"

This comprehensive approach must take in more than other health factors. Perhaps more than any other disease, HIV/AIDS will not be contained as long as it is regarded as a health issue and not placed within the overall context of development. According to Jean-Louis Lamboray of the World Bank: "If we take a narrow view of the threat of HIV and STDs, we will not achieve any effect [8]." James Makumbi, Ugandan Minister of Health, suggests that all aspects of government must be involved: "The overall effect of the disease is such that no one ministry can handle it [9]."

Broadening the response to HIV/AIDS has short-term as well as long-term advantages. In most governments the ministry of health has much less influence than ministries of finance or industry. Even where the virus is not widespread, involving those ministries at an early stage gives the health ministry greater backing. Yet when drawing up HIV/AIDS strategies, relatively few governments involve other ministries, or indeed the business community or NGOs. Two notable exceptions are Thailand and Uganda, where the NACP answers directly to the head of government, and committee members include representatives of health, education and finance ministries.

In the words of Michael Merson, director of GPA, "The first challenge is for those... leaders who have not yet done so, to give their fullest political commitment to the fight against

Health centre in India. People's health is linked to their social and economic circumstances. HIV/AIDS cannot be tackled in isolation from other aspects of development.

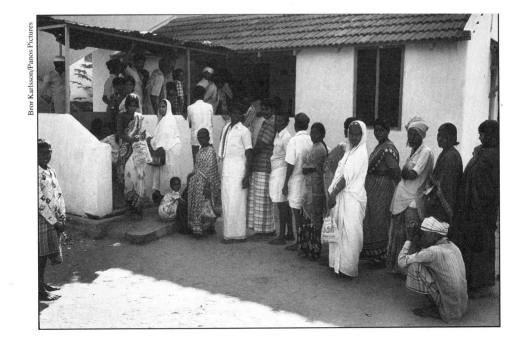

Bror Karlsson/Panos Pictures

"The development process itself is threatened"

AIDS....Prevention and care programmes simply cannot succeed unless they receive the wholehearted support and backing of the very highest levels of government. AIDS is essentially a sexually transmitted disease and yes, sensitivities abound. But top-level political commitment opens minds and doors. It removes obstacles to action by those who have the will and know-how to move against the pandemic [10]."

One of the faults of development planning has been the tendency to think in sectors; HIV/AIDS is a classic example of a problem which needs an integrated approach. Broad-based NACPs are more likely to encourage a comprehensive response to the epidemic and to address issues of poverty and powerlessness. By involving different sectors and areas of expertise in HIV/AIDS planning, policymaking can benefit from a two-way process. For example, finance ministries can give their input and support to HIV/AIDS activities, while HIV/AIDS expertise can influence decisionmaking in finance and other sectors. Similarly, involving relevant development NGOs and organisations in NACPs should lead to integration of activities rather than duplication, and so potential resentment from agencies working in other areas of development can be avoided. Since many health care, agricultural, nutrition, education and income generation programmes will have an impact on the HIV/AIDS epidemic, the question of how to allocate funds does not necessarily have to break down into an either/or situation, while HIV/AIDS programmes can be designed and funded in a way that contributes to the general strengthening of other services rather than detracts from them.

The need to recognise the challenge HIV/AIDS poses to development was summed up by Michael Merson when he said, "All sectors of life are threatened. So is the development process itself....While developing countries have shown resourcefulness in meeting many of their needs to date...[they] cannot possibly shoulder alone all the AIDS-related funding needs in the coming decade.....It is particularly important to increase overall development assistance, not only to alleviate the pandemic's impact on all sectors of the economy, but also to diminish poverty, because poverty makes countries vulnerable to the further spread of [the disease]....AIDS is an unprecedented challenge....each and every one of us has a direct stake in averting the human, social and economic cost of [its] further spread [11]."

Summary

Causes

- **HIV/AIDS is only secondarily a health problem** The epidemic is driven by social and economic factors which make some individuals more vulnerable to infection.
- **Poverty fuels the spread of HIV/AIDS** Communities struggling with inadequate health facilities, high levels of illiteracy and low incomes are often more at risk.
- **Patterns of HIV infection reflect inequality between the sexes** Women's lower social and economic status often makes them less able to protect themselves against the risk of infection.
- **The long incubation period of HIV/AIDS encourages its spread** Because the true costs of the epidemic remain hidden for some time, political action and behaviour change can be difficult to achieve in the early stages.

Predicting the future

- **In most countries the epidemic is in an early stage** The second stage of the epidemic, when significant numbers fall ill, may not be apparent until the mid-1990s or the end of the century.
- **Mortality rates will rise** Demographic models predict adult and under-five mortality will rise. Life expectancies will fall.
- **Population growth will slow** Populations will continue to grow, although at a slower rate than before. Population decline is unlikely.
- **The impact on fertility is uncertain** Increased child mortality may be matched by increasing numbers of births.
- **Overall dependency ratios may not change** But the death of many young and middle-aged adults will place the burden of dependency more heavily on younger, less skilled members of the labour force.

The social cost

- **The initial focus of the epidemic will be the household** Because transmission is predominantly through sexual intercourse, and from mother to child, often more than one household member will contract the disease.
- **Changes in household structure will result** The roles of grandparents and other relatives, parents and children will change in response to illness and death. Labour and income will be lost.
- **The traditional coping mechanisms of the wider community will come under increasing strain** The burden of caring for the sick, taking in orphans and compensating for lost labour will outweigh the abilities of communities to cope.
- **Children will suffer physical and psychological deprivation** Many children will be orphaned, many will be drawn out of school to look after parents or take on work, many will suffer impoverishment and poor nutrition.
- **Some traditional patterns of behaviour may alter as a result of the epidemic** Both social and economic relationships within communities may break down or be adapted as a result of attempts to prevent the spread of HIV/AIDS or cope with its impact.

The economic cost

- **The disease may lead to overall labour shortages in rural areas** This has implications for nutrition, food production and security at local and national levels.
- **Countries and institutions dependent on relatively few skilled and managerial staff face long-term difficulties** There is evidence that in certain areas, the epidemic has had a disproportionate effect on more skilled and educated male workers.

- **The epidemic may lead to a younger, less experienced workforce** Large numbers of people dying in adulthood will mean a significant loss of more experienced workers.
- **HIV/AIDS leads to lowered productivity** Once symptoms develop, the illness is characterised by bouts of ill health, resulting in loss of labour. Absenteeism also results from people having to care for the ill.
- **Exports and foreign exchange may decline** The epidemic may result in reduced domestic production, fewer goods to export, fewer remittances from migrants abroad.

Conclusions

- **Medical research should be complemented by socio-economic research** Little is understood about the patterns of sexual behaviour and other social and cultural practices which may contribute to the spread of the disease.
- **Specific population groups must be targeted for education** Mass awareness campaigns need to be complemented by interventions tailored for specific groups.
- **STD treatment should be made a priority** Untreated STDs greatly facilitate the spread of HIV/AIDS.
- **Existing health structures need to be strengthened** HIV/AIDS cannot be tackled in isolation from other health issues.
- **Money should be directed towards HIV/AIDS care and treatment** Care is part of prevention. Failure to treat is not only unethical, but it adds to the stigma of the disease and encourages its spread.
- **Development agencies need to take account of the implications of HIV/AIDS in all their activities** Development which improves people's social and economic conditions and reduces dependence on practices such as migration and prostitution will **reduce transmission** of the disease. Policies which take account of the likely effects of the disease can **reduce the impact.**
- **Communities develop and adapt their own coping mechanisms** External agencies should support and assist this process.
- **Some new development initiatives may be necessary** Credit schemes, for example, may need to be rethought in areas with high levels of HIV/AIDS.
- **Research into the agricultural impact is necessary** Research and development is needed, for example, on crops which require less labour but are nutritious; cultivation practices which are less labour-intensive; and labour-saving appropriate technologies.
- **Improvement in women's social and economic status is a prerequisite for increasing their ability to protect themselves and their children from the epidemic**
- **Education and training policies need to take account of the impact of the epidemic**
- **Economic plans need to take account of possible changes in the labour supply**
- **Mechanisms for delivery of money and expertise to fight HIV/AIDS at all levels must be improved** Not only funds but management or technical support may be needed.
- **Whatever the extent of HIV infection in the population, governments need to undertake extensive awareness and education programmes** Low rates of infection provide an opportunity to prevent a serious epidemic; high rates of infection require urgent measures.
- **Whatever the extent of HIV infection in the population, governments need to provide an integrated response to the epidemic** National AIDS Control Programmes must be strengthened. Finance and education ministries must be involved.

References

INTRODUCTION

1. Panos convened the Talloires Consultation in collaboration with the American Foundation for AIDS Research (AMFAR), the Norwegian Red Cross, the Swedish International Development Authority (SIDA) and WHO.
2. WHO Press Release WHO/28, 1 May 1992.
3. Viravaidya, M and others, "The economic impact of AIDS on Thailand", October 1991.

CHAPTER 1

1. *Morbidity and Mortality Weekly Report*, 5 June 1981, Vol 30, No 21, pp250-252; Gottleib, M and others, *New England Journal of Medicine*, 10 December 1981, Vol 305, No 24, pp1425-1431.
2. *The Current Global Situation of the HIV/AIDS Pandemic*, WHO Global Programme on AIDS, Geneva, July 1992.
3. WHO Press Release, WHO/9, 12 February 1992.
4. WHO diagram, JC/TRANS/92.
5. Unless otherwise referenced, statistics in this and following paragraphs are from *Current and Future Dimensions of the HIV/AIDS Pandemic: a capsule summary*, WHO, Geneva, January 1992.
6. *Asian Wall Street Journal*, 3 September 1990, quoted in *AIDS Newsletter*, 1990/768.
7. Wawer, M J and others, "Geographic and community distribution of HIV-1 infection in rural Rakai district, Uganda", *Abstracts of VIth International Conference on AIDS,* San Francisco, 1990, FC 606.
8. Over, M and Piot, P, "HIV infection and sexually transmitted diseases", in Jamison, D and Mosley, W (eds), *Disease Control Priorities in Developing Countries*, World Bank, forthcoming.
9. Information from Martin Donoghoe, Centre for Research on Drug and Health Behaviour, London, UK, August 1992.
10. Over, M and Piot, P, op. cit.
11. Pepin, J and others, "The interaction between HIV infection and other sexually transmitted diseases: an opportunity for intervention", *AIDS*, 1989, Vol 3, pp3-9.
12. Laga, M and others, "Non-ulcerative sexually transmitted diseases (STD) as risk factors for HIV infection", *Abstracts of VIth International Conference on AIDS*, San Francisco, 1990, ThC97; Ombette, J and others, "Presence of HIV among men and women with *H. ducreyi* and *Neisseria gonorrhoeae* infection in Nairobi, Kenya", *Abstracts of VIth International Conference on AIDS*, San Francisco, 1990, ThC572.
13. Arya, O and Bennett, F, "Role of the medical auxiliary in the control of sexually transmitted disease in a developing country", *British Journal of Venereal*

Diseases, 1976, Vol 52, pp116-121.

14. Information from André Mehens, WHO.

15. WHO Features, December 1990, No 152.

16. Potts, M and others, "Slowing the spread of human immunodeficiency virus in developing countries", *Lancet*, 1991, Vol 338, pp608-613; European Study Group on Heterosexual Transmission of HIV, "Comparison of female to male and male to female transmission of HIV in 563 stable couples" *British Medical Journal*, 1992, Vol 304, pp809-813.

17. "Contraceptive Methods and Human Immunodeficiency Virus (HIV)", WHO/SPA/INF/87.9, WHO, Geneva, 1987.

18. Schoepf, B, "Women, AIDS and economic crisis in Central Africa", *Canadian Journal of African Studies*, 1988, Vol 22, pp625-644; Brown, R C and others, "Vaginal Inflammation in Africa", *New England Journal of Medicine*, 1992, Vol 326, p572.

19. "Anatomy as Destiny: Young Women and HIV—age as an independent variable in the acquisition of HIV infection", unpublished paper, UNDP.

20. Ibid.

21. Prual, A and others, "Sexual behaviour, AIDS and poverty in sub-Saharan Africa", *International Journal of STD and AIDS*, 1991, Vol 2, pp1-9.

22. Cameron, W and others, "Female to male transmission of human immunodeficiency virus type 1: risk factors for seroconversion in men", *New England Journal of Medicine*, 1989, Vol 321, pp403-407.

23. De Vincenzi, I and Ancelle-Park, R, "Heterosexual transmission of HIV: a European study", *Abstracts of Vth International Conference on AIDS*, Montreal, 1989, ThAO20.

24. Johnson, A and Laga, M, "Heterosexual transmission of HIV", *AIDS*, 1988, Vol 2, ppS49-S56.

25. From information supplied by Brook Advisory Centre, London, 1992.

26. Sanders, S and Sambo, A, "AIDS in Africa: the implications of economic recession and structural adjustment", *Health Policy and Planning*, 1991, Vol 6, pp157-162.

27. Interview, August 1992.

28. *Human Development Report 1992*, UNDP, Table 16.

29. Communication with Panos, July 1992; see also, for a fuller discussion of women and HIV/AIDS, *Triple Jeopardy: women and AIDS*, Panos, London, 1990.

30. Allen, S and others, "Human immunodeficiency virus infection in urban Rwanda", *Journal of the American Medical Association*, 1991, Vol 266, pp1657-1663.

31. Kreiss, J K and others, "AIDS virus infection in Nairobi prostitutes", *New England Journal of Medicine*, 1986, Vol 314, pp414-418.

32. Bhave, G and others, "HIV sero surveillance in promiscuous females of Bombay, India", *Abstracts of VIth International Conference on AIDS*, San Francisco, 1990, FC 612.

33. Anderson, R M and others, "The potential demographic and economic impact of AIDS in sub-Saharan Africa", report to Overseas Development Administration, London, March 1991.

34. Schoepf, B, "Women, AIDS and economic crisis in Central Africa", *Canadian Journal of African Studies*, 1988, Vol 22, pp625-644.

35. Merson, M, address to VIIIth International Conference on AIDS, Amsterdam, 1992.

36. A minority of researchers believe that HIV does not lead to AIDS; see Duesberg,

P, "Human immunodeficiency virus and acquired immunodeficiency syndrome: correlation but not causation", *Proceedings of the National Academy of Science USA*, 1989, Vol 86, pp755-764.

37. See Piot, P and others, "The global epidemiology of HIV infection: continuity, heterogeneity and change", *Journal of Acquired Immune Deficiency Syndromes*, 1990, Vol 3, pp403-412.

38. Muller, O and others, "AIDS in Africa", *New England Journal of Medicine*, 1991, Vol 324, pp847-8; Brindle, R and others, *Abstracts of VIth International Conference on AIDS in Africa*, Dakar, 1991, WA 199; *AIDS Analysis Africa*, November/December 1991.

39. "Acquired Immunodeficiency Syndrome (AIDS): interim proposal for a WHO staging system for HIV infection and disease", *Weekly Epidemiological Record*, 20 July 1990, pp221-224.

40. Peckham, C and Newell, M-L, "HIV infection in mothers and babies", *AIDS Care*, 1990, Vol 2, pp205-211; Tovo, P and others, "Prognostic factors and survival in children with perinatal HIV-1 infection", *Lancet*, 1992, Vol 339, pp1249-1253.

41. Krivine, A and others, "HIV replication during the first weeks of life", *Lancet*, 1992, Vol 339, pp1187-1189; Futh, L and others, "Mode of delivery in HIV-1 infected women", *Lancet*, 1992, Vol 339, p1603.

42. Van de Perre, P and others, "Postnatal transmission of Human Immunodeficiency Virus Type 1 from mother to infant", *New England Journal of Medicine*, 1992, Vol 326, pp643-644; see also *Abstracts of VIIIth International Conference on AIDS*, Amsterdam, 1992, ThC 1520-ThC 1524.

43. WHO Press Release WHO/30, 4 May 1992.

44. See *Abstracts of VIIIth International Conference on AIDS*, Amsterdam, 1992, WeC 1063-WeC 1067.

45. Hamilton, J and others, "A controlled trial of early versus late treatment with zidovudine in symptomatic HIV infection. Results of the veterans affairs cooperative study", *New England Journal of Medicine*, 1992, Vol 326, pp437-443; Neil, M and others, "The effects of survival of early treatment of Human Immunodeficiency Virus infection", *New England Journal of Medicine*, 1992, Vol 326, pp1037-1042.

46. Larson, A, "Social context of HIV transmission in Africa: historical and cultural bases of East and Central Africa sexual relations", *Review of Infectious Diseases*, 1989, Vol 11, pp716-31; Larson, A, "The Social Context of HIV Transmission in Africa", Health Transition Centre Working Paper 1, Australian National University; Gopalan, C, *NFI Bulletin*, 1992, Vol 13, pp1-3, quoted in *AIDS Newsletter*, 1992/363.

47. This paragraph derives from Zwi, A and Cabral, A, "Identifying 'high risk situations' for preventing AIDS", *British Medical Journal*, 1991, Vol 303, pp1527-1529.

48. Viravaidya, M and others, "The economic impact of AIDS on Thailand", October 1991.

49. For further discussion see Hunt, C, "Migrant labour and sexually transmitted disease: AIDS in Africa", *Journal of Health and Social Behavior*, 1989, Vol 30, pp353-373.

50. See, for example, Malamba, S and others, *Abstracts of VIth International Conference on AIDS in Africa*, Dakar, 1991, MA 244; Van de Perre, P and others, "HIV antibodies in a remote rural area in Rwanda, Central Africa: an analysis of potential risk factors for HIV seropositivity", *AIDS*, 1987, Vol 1, pp213-215.

CHAPTER 2

1. Prediction of over 100 million infections made by Gobal AIDS Policy Coalition, Harvard University; other figures in this paragraph from *Current and Future Dimensions of the HIV/AIDS Pandemic: a capsule summary, January 1992*, WHO.
2. *The State of World Population 1991*, UNFPA.
3. *Human Development Report 1992*, UNDP.
4. *The Health of Adults in the Developing World*, World Bank, May 1991.
5. For a summary of the main models see *The AIDS Epidemic and its Demographic Consequences*, ST/ESA/SER.A/119, UN/WHO, 1991. Critiques of models are to be found in Becker, C, "The demo-economic impact of the AIDS pandemic in sub-Saharan Africa", *World Development*, 1990, Vol 18, pp1599-1619; and Over, M and Piot, P, "HIV infection and sexually transmitted diseases", in Jamison, D and Mosley, W (eds), *Disease Control Priorities in Developing Countries*, World Bank, forthcoming.
6. See, for example, Anderson, R and others, "The potential demographic and economic impact of AIDS in sub-Saharan Africa", report to Overseas Development Administration, London, March 1991.
7. Chin, J, "Epidemiology: current and future dimensions of the HIV/AIDS pandemic in women and children", *Lancet*, 1990, Vol 336, pp221-224.
8. Becker, C, "The demo-economic impact of the AIDS pandemic in sub-Saharan Africa", *World Development*, 1990, Vol 18, p 1610.
9. "Projecting the demographic impact of the HIV/AIDS pandemic", WHO document, GPA/GMC(1)91.8.
10. Bulatao, R, "The Bulatao approach: projecting the demographic impact of the HIV epidemic using standard parameters", in *The AIDS Epidemic and its Demographic Consequences*, op. cit.
11. Anderson, R and others, op. cit.
12. "Children and AIDS: an impending calamity", UNICEF, New York, 1990.
13. Preble, E A, "Impact of HIV/AIDS on African children", *Social Science and Medicine*, 1990, Vol 31, pp671-680.
14. Chin, J, op. cit.
15. "Projecting the demographic impact of the HIV/AIDS pandemic", op. cit.
16. See, for example, Liomba, G and others, "Mortality experience in children of HIV-1 infected mothers in Malawi", *Abstracts of VIIIth International Conference on AIDS*, Amsterdam, 1992, PoC 4238.
17. Latter two points from Becker, C, op. cit.
18. Quotes from Ankrah, E M, "AIDS: socio-economic decline and health. A double crisis for the African woman", in press.
19. Interview with Jane Rowley, Imperial College, London, August 1992.
20. de Cock, K and others, "Stability of HIV infection prevalence over 10 years in a rural population of Zaire", *Abstracts of IIIrd International Conference on AIDS*, Washington, 1987, WP 43.
21. See, for example, *Abstracts of VIIIth International Conference on AIDS*, Amsterdam, 1992, PoC 4016, and PoC 4019.
22. Rowley, J and others, "Reducing the spread of HIV infection in sub-Saharan Africa: some demographic and economic implications", *AIDS*, 1990, Vol 4, pp47-56.
23. Adapted from Over, M and Piot, P, "HIV infection and sexually transmitted diseases", op. cit.

24. Anderson, R and others, op. cit.
25. Way, P O and Stanecki, K, "The Demographic Impact of an AIDS epidemic on an African country: application of the IWG AIDS model", US Bureau of the Census, CIR Staff Paper No 58, 1991.
26. Ibid.
27. Viravaidya, M and others, "The economic impact of AIDS on Thailand", October 1991.
28. Over, M and Piot, P, op. cit.
29. See "The HIV catch-22", *Lancet*, 1991, Vol 337, P843.
30. Ruan, F F, *Sex in China*, Plenum Press, New York/London, 1991; Roddy, R E and others, "Genital ulcers in women", *Lancet*, 1989, Vol 334, pp558-559.
31. Address at VIth International Conference on AIDS, San Francisco, 1990.
32. Chin, J and others, "Projections of HIV infections and AIDS cases to the year 2000", *Bulletin of the World Health Organization*, 1990, Vol 68, pp1-11.
33. *Current and Future Dimensions of the HIV/AIDS Pandemic: a capsule summary*, WHO, Geneva, January 1992.

CHAPTER 3

1. Cameron, C and Tarantola, D, "The costs of AIDS care in the world", *Abstracts of the VIIIth International Conference on AIDS*, Amsterdam, 1992, WeC 1038.
2. Calculated from data in *Human Development Report 1992*, UNDP.
3. *World Drug Situation*, Action Programme on Essential Drugs, WHO, Geneva, 1988, quoted in Foster, S, "Affordable clinical care for HIV-related opportunistic infections in developing countries", paper presented at WHO Informal Consultation on Opportunistic Infections in Developing Countries, September 1989.
4. Foster, S and others, *Supply and Use of Essential Drugs in sub-Saharan Africa: issues and possible solutions*, Africa Health Policy Background Paper, Washington DC, World Bank, 1989, quoted in Foster, S, "Affordable clinical care for HIV- related opportunistic infections in developing countries", op. cit.
5. *Human Development Report 1992*, UNDP.
6. Ibid.
7. Information from ActionAid, Nepal, July 1992.
8. An analysis of methodology in calculating the costs of HIV/AIDS can be found in Over, M and others, "Guidelines for rapid estimation of the direct and indirect costs of HIV infection in a developing country", *Health Policy*, 1989, Vol 11, pp169-186.
9. Hellinger, Fred J, "Forecasts of the medical care costs of the HIV epidemic in the United States: 1992-1995", paper presented at *VIIIth International Conference on AIDS*, Amsterdam, 1992.
10. Over, M and others, "Guidelines for rapid estimation of the direct and indirect costs of HIV infection in a developing country", op. cit.
11. Foster, S, "Affordable clinical care for HIV-related opportunistic infections in developing countries", op. cit.
12. Viravaidya, M and others, "The economic impact of AIDS on Thailand", October 1991.
13. Quinn, T and others, "AIDS in the Americas: a public health priority for the region", *AIDS*, 1990, Vol 4, pp709-724.
14. Studies quoted in Hanson, K, "The Economic Impact of AIDS: an assessment of the available evidence", report submitted to Global Programme on AIDS, March 1992.

15. Esteves, R and others, "The direct costs of hospital care of AIDS patients in Brazil", *Abstracts of VIIIth International Conference on AIDS*, Amsterdam, 1992, WeC 1035; see also Cordeiro, H, "Medical costs of HIV and AIDS in Brazil", in Fleming, A and others (eds), *The Global Impact of AIDS*, New York, 1988, gives a figure of $21,500 for annual medical costs in Brazil.

16. Hellinger, Fred J, op. cit.

17. Foster, S, "Affordable clinical care for HIV-related opportunistic infections in developing countries", op. cit.

18. Viravaidya, M and others, op. cit.

19. Hassig, S and others, "An analysis of the economic impact of HIV infection among patients at Mama Yemo Hospital, Kinshasa, Zaire", *AIDS*, 1990, Vol 4, pp883-887.

20. Interview with Susan Foster, December 1991.

21. Loemba, H and others, "Tuberculosis associated HIV in Congo", *Abstracts of VIIIth International Conference on AIDS*, Amsterdam, 1992, PuB 7319.

22. Green, J and others, "AIDS and tuberculosis in New York Hospitals", *Abstracts of VIIIth International Conference on AIDS*, Amsterdam, 1992, PuC 8095.

23. Foster, S, *Study of Economic Aspects of Adult Illness in Zambia, Progress Report no. 3*, London School of Hygiene and Tropical Medicine, 1991.

24. Speech by President Museveni at the VIIth International Conference on AIDS, Florence, June 1991.

25. Cruz, M and others, "Experience at the care clinic for HIV seropositive patients", *Abstracts of VIIIth International Conference on AIDS*, Amsterdam, 1992, PuB 7128.

26. Gray, A, *Economic Aspects of AIDS and HIV Infection in the UK*, London School of Hygiene and Tropical Medicine, 1991.

27. Hassig, S and others, op. cit.

28. Foster, S and others, "Costs of treatment for HIV disease at a district hospital in Zambia", *Abstracts of VIIIth International Conference on AIDS*, Amsterdam, 1992, PoD 5769.

29. N'Galy, B and others, "Obstacles to the optimal management of HIV infection/AIDS in Africa", *Journal of Acquired Immune Deficiency Syndromes*, 1990, Vol 3, pp430-437.

30. Communication from Elizabeth Ngugi, University of Niarobi, July 1992.

31. Foster, S, *Study of Economic Aspects of Adult Illness in Zambia, Progress Report no. 3*, op. cit.

32. Private communication with Susan Foster, August 1992.

33. O'Donahue, M, "The impact of AIDS/HIV on hospitals and health services", *Is AIDS a Development Issue?*, UK NGO AIDS Consortium for the Third World, London, 1990.

34. Ngcongco, V N, presentation at VIth International Conference on AIDS, San Francisco, 1990.

35. Interview with Susan Foster, December 1992.

36. Ainsworth, M and Over, M, "The economic impact of AIDS: shocks, responses and outcomes", World Bank, Africa Technical Department: Population, Health and Nutrition Division, Technical Working Paper No 1, June 1992, pp13-14. The authors note that these figures should be treated with caution.

37. *Business Day*, Johannesburg, 1990.

38. Shephard, D and others, "Costs of AIDS care in Rwanda", *Abstracts of VIIIth International Conference on AIDS*, Amsterdam, 1992, PoD 5505.

39. Whiteside, A, "AIDS in Zimbabwe: An Assessment", The Southern Africa

Foundation for Economic Research, Harare, 1991, p32.

40. Anderson, R and others, "The potential demographic and economic impact of AIDS in sub-Saharan Africa", report to Overseas Development Administration, London, March 1991, Chapter 5, p7

41. *1991 World Health Statistics Annual*, WHO, Geneva, 1992, p23.

42. Interview with Paul Nunn, August 1992.

43. Narain, J, Raviglione, M and Kochi, A, *HIV-associated Tuberculosis in Developing Countries: Epidemiology and Strategies for Prevention*, WHO, Geneva, WHO/TB/92.166.

44. Schuber, M et al, "An estimate of the future size of the tuberculosis problem in sub-Saharan Africa resulting from HIV infection", *Tubercle and Lung Disease*, No 73, 1992, ppS2-S8.

45. Interview with Mario Raviglione of WHO, August 1992.

46. Interview with Ishwar Gilada, Indian Health Association, August 1992.

47. See, for example, Cooper, D A, "The efficacy and safety of zidovudine therapy in early asymptomatic HIV infection", *Abstracts of the VIIIth International Conference on AIDS*, Amsterdam, 1992, PoB 3718.

48. Hellinger, F J, op. cit.

49. Kimball, A and others, *The Feasibility of Providing AZT Through National AIDS Programs in Latin America: What would it cost?*, PAHO, 1990.

50. Ibid.

51. Panos calculation.

CHAPTER 4

1. Devereux, S and Eele, G, "The social and economic impact of AIDS in East and Central Africa", Food Studies Group, Oxford University, May 1991, p13.

2. McGuire, J F, "AIDS: the community-based response", *AIDS*, 1989, Vol 3, Suppl 1, pS279.

3. Hunter, S, "Orphans as a window on the AIDS epidemic in sub-Saharan Africa: initial results and implications of a study in Uganda", *Social Science and Medicine*, 1990, Vol 31(6), pp681-690, quoted in Devereux, S and Eele, G, op. cit.

4. Barnett, A and Blaikie, P, *AIDS in Africa: its present and future impact*, Belhaven Press, London, 1992, pp111-112.

5. Ankrah, E M and others, "The impact of AIDS on urban families: an assessment of needs", *Abstracts of VIth International Conference on AIDS in Africa*, Dakar, 1991, WA 251.

6. Feuerstein, M-T and Lovel, H, "Seeing light at the end of the tunnel: positive and negative implications and community responses to the challenge of HIV infection and AIDS", *Community Development Journal*, July 1989, Vol 24, No 3, pp169-170.

7. Devereux, S and Eele, G, op. cit., p21.

8. Bond, G and Vincent, J, "Living on the edge: structural adjustment in the context of AIDS", quoted in Devereux, S and Eele, G, op. cit.

9. Information from "Responding to AIDS in East Africa: policy and proposals for action", ACORD, 16 June 1992.

10. Hunter, S, op. cit.

11. For a fuller discussion of such implications, see van de Walle, E, "The social impact of AIDS in sub-Saharan Africa", *The Millbank Quarterly*, 1990, Vol 68, Suppl 1, pp10-32.

12. Mouli, V C, "Trends in the responses of communities", paper presented at the

VIIIth International Conference on AIDS, Amsterdam, 1992.

13.   Presentation by Theresa Kaijage of WAMATA to the UK All-Party Parliamentary Group on AIDS, 14 May 1991.

14.   Ibid.

15.   Norse, D, "Socio-economic impact of AIDS on food production in east Africa", paper presented at VIIth International Conference on AIDS, Florence, June 1991.

16.   Pryer, J, "When breadwinners fall ill: preliminary findings from a case study in Bangladesh", *IDS Bulletin*, April 1989, Vol 20, No 2, pp49-57.

17.   *Analyse de la situation des enfants et des femmes au Congo*, UNICEF, Document de travail, Brazzaville, May 1991.

18.   Mukoyogo, M C and Williams, G, *AIDS Orphans—a community perspective from Tanzania: strategies for hope No 5*, ActionAid, London, 1991.

19.   Preble, E and Foumbi, J, "The African family and AIDS: a current look at the epidemic", *AIDS*, 1991, Vol 5, Suppl 2, ppS265-S269.

20.   Presentation by Theresa Kaijage of WAMATA to the UK All-Party Parliamentary Group on AIDS, 14 May 1991.

21.   Foster, S, *Study of Economic Aspects of Adult Illness in Zambia*, London School of Hygiene and Tropical Medicine, update on research activities, Zambia, August 1991.

22.   Feachem, R G A and others (eds), *The Health of Adults in the Developing World*, Oxford University Press for the World Bank, New York, 1991.

23.   "Children and AIDS: an impending calamity", UNICEF, New York, 1990.

24.   "Children orphaned by HIV in Africa", paper presented by James Ssekiwanuka, SCF Uganda, at Institute of Child Health, London, October 1991.

25.   Information from "Responding to AIDS in East Africa: policy and proposals for action", ACORD, 16 June 1992.

26.   Dunn, A and Hunter, S, "Uganda, AIDS and families", *Is AIDS a development issue?*, UK NGO AIDS Consortium for the Third World, London 1989.

27.   Paper prepared for Panos by Sheldon Shaeffer of the International Institute for Educational Planning, Paris, June 1992.

28.   Barnett, A and Blaikie, P, *AIDS in Africa*, op. cit.

29.   Barnett, A and Blaikie P, *AIDS Analysis Africa, Southern Africa Edition*, October/November 1991.

30.   Feuerstein, M-T and Lovel, H, op. cit, p164.

31.   Ibid, p169.

32.   Presentation by Theresa Kaijage of WAMATA to the UK All-Party Parliamentary Group on AIDS, 14 May 1991.

33.   Preble, E A, "Impact of HIV/AIDS on African children", *Social Science and Medicine*, 1990, Vol 6, pp671-680.

34.   *AIDS Analysis Africa*, July/August 1991.

35.   Viravaidya, M and others, "The economic impact of AIDS in Thailand", October 1991.

36.   "Children orphaned by HIV in Africa", op. cit.

37.   Lwanga, J S, "Children whose parents die of AIDS", *Abstracts of VIth International Conference on AIDS in Africa*, Dakar, 1991, WTR 308.

38.   *AIDS: New Challenges in Development Cooperation*, NORAD, Oslo, 1991, p30.

39.   "Tanzania AIDS assessment and planning study", World Bank, 1991, p72.

40.   Personal communication.

41.   "Tanzania AIDS assessment and planning study", op. cit., p73.

42.   Matovu, N K and others, "A study of behaviour change, community depression and community coping mechanisms in five selected villages in Kirumba

sub-county, Rakai district", Makerere University, Kampala, February 1992.
43. Reported in *The Journal of Infectious Diseases*, March 1992.

CHAPTER 5

1. Anderson, R and others, "The potential demographic and economic impact of AIDS in sub-Saharan Africa", report to Overseas Development Administration, London, March 1991.
2. *AIDS Analysis Africa*, November/December 1991.
3. *Southern African Economist*, April/May 1992.
4. Ryder, R and others, "Heterosexual transmission of HIV-1 among employees and their spouses at two large businesses in Zaire", *AIDS*, 1990, Vol 8, pp725-732; Hassig, S and others, "An analysis of the economic impact of HIV infection among patients at Mama Yemo Hospital, Kinshasa, Zaire", *AIDS*, 1990, Vol 4, pp883-887.
5. Bugingo, G and others, "Etude sur la séropositivité liée à l'infection au virus de l'immunodéficience humaine au Rwanda", *Revue Médicale Rwandaise*, 1988, Vol 20, pp37- 42, quoted in Over, M and Piot, P, "HIV infection and sexually transmitted diseases", in Jamison, D and Mosley, W (eds), *Disease Control Priorities in Developing Countries*, World Bank, forthcoming.
6. Melbye, M and others, "Evidence for heterosexual transmission and clinical manifestations of human immunodeficiency virus infection and related conditions in Lusaka, Zambia", *Lancet*, 1986, Vol 328, pp1113-1115.
7. Allen, S and others, "Human Immunodeficiency Virus infection in urban Rwanda", *Journal of the American Medical Association*, 1991, Vol 266, No 12, pp1657-1663.
8. Ryder, R and others, op. cit.
9. *Financial Gazette*, Harare, 30 November 1990.
10. *National Mirror*, Lusaka, 6 April 1991.
11. Economist Intelligence Unit, 1992, quoted in *Financial Times*, London, 23 January 1992.
12. See, for example, Lauria, L M and others, "The changing of AIDS epidemiology in Rio de Janeiro", *Abstracts of VIIIth International Conference on AIDS*, Amsterdam, 1992, PoC 4049.
13. *Financial Gazette*, op. cit.
14. *National Mirror*, op. cit.
15. "AIDS news is not good, not catastrophic", *Finance Week*, June 27-July 3 1991, South Africa, p49.
16. See, for example, Najera, J and others, "Health sector priorities review: malaria", in Jamison, D and Mosley, W (eds), op. cit.
17. Information from confidential correspondence, 1991.
18. Becker, C, "The demo-economic impact of the AIDS pandemic in sub-Saharan Africa", *World Development*, 1990, Vol 18, No 12, pp1599-1619.
19. Information from confidential correspondence, 1991.
20. *South*, June/July 1991.
21. Viravaidya, M and others, "The economic impact of AIDS on Thailand", October 1991.
22. Whiteside, A, "HIV infection and AIDS in Zimbabwe: an assessment", Southern Africa Foundation for Economic Research, Harare, 1991; "The Money Programme: The Wasting of Africa", BBC2 Television, UK, 31 May 1992
23. Ponnighaus, J M and Oxborrow, S M, "Construction projects and spread of HIV", *Lancet*, 1990, Vol 336, p1198.

24. *South*, op. cit.
25. *National Mirror*, op. cit.
26. *AIDS Analysis Africa*, September/October 1991.
27. *Southern African Economist*, April/May 1992.
28. Ibid.
29. Ibid.
30. Interview, July 1992.
31. For examples, see *The Third Epidemic; repercussions of the fear of AIDS*, Panos, London, 1990, Chapter 5.
32. Whiteside, A, op. cit., pp36-37.
33. *Statement from the Consultation on AIDS and the Workplace*, WHO/ILO, Geneva, 27-29 June 1988, WHO/GPA/INF/88.7.
34. Whiteside, A, op. cit.
35. Whiteside, A, op. cit., pp39-40.
36. *National Mirror*, op. cit.
37. For further discussion of the response of the commercial sector to HIV/AIDS see *The Third Epidemic: repercussions of the fear of AIDS*, op. cit.
38. *Business Day*, Johannesburg, 19 October 1990.
39. Report to Panos by Juan Carlos Tinant, Argentinian Family Planning Association, 1992.
40. Jespersen, E, unpublished UNICEF document quoted in Sanders, D and Sambo, A, "AIDS in Africa: the implications of economic recession and structural adjustment", *Health Policy and Planning*, 1991, Vol 6(2), pp157-165.
41. Knight, V C, "AIDS threatens insurance industry", *Africa South*, July/August 1990, p12.
42. Van Niftrik, J, "Insurance industry exposure", *AIDS Analysis Africa, Southern Africa Edition*, Vol 2, No 3, October/November 1991, p3.
43. Van Niftrik, J, "Alarming rise in SA insurance claims", *AIDS Analysis Africa, Southern Africa Edition*, Vol 2, No 6, April/May 1992, p7.
44. Whiteside, A, op. cit., p25.
45. "The Money Programme: The Wasting of Africa", BBC2 Television, UK, 31 May 1992.

CHAPTER 6

1. Norse, D, "Socio-economic impact of AIDS on food production in East Africa", paper presented at VIIth International Conference on AIDS, Florence, June 1991.
2. Wawer, M and others, "Dynamics of spread of HIV-1 infection in a rural district of Uganda", *British Medical Journal*, 1991, Vol 303, pp1303-1306; Killewo, J and others, "Prevalence of HIV-1 infection in the Kagera region of Tanzania: a population-based study", *AIDS*, 1990, Vol 4, pp1081-1085.
3. Mutembei, I, "AIDS and development: the survey of AIDS deaths and social economic impact in Tanzania", *Abstracts of VIth International Conference on AIDS in Africa*, Dakar, 1991, TO 117.
4. *World Development Report 1992—Development and the Environment*, Oxford University Press for the World Bank.
5. United States Department of Agriculture, International Economics Division of the Statistical Service, *World Food Aid Needs and Availabilities*, Washington DC, March 1981, quoted in Abel, N and others, "The impact of AIDS on food production systems in East and Central Africa over the next ten years: a programmatic paper" in Fleming, A and others, *The Global Impact of AIDS*, Alan R Liss Inc, London, 1988.

6. *Human Development Report 1992*, UNDP, Table 4.
7. For a fuller discussion of patterns of labour in Africa and divisions by sex and age, see Swindell, K, *Farm Labour*, Cambridge University Press, African Society Today series, Cambridge, 1985, Chapter 1.
8. "Malawi Food Security Report", No 8151-MAI, 1989, unpublished World Bank report.
9. Norse, D, op. cit.
10. Chipande, G H R, "Socio-economic aspects of female-headed households and rural development efforts, with special reference to the Phalombe area of Malawi", paper presented at Workshop on Rural Development Strategies and Programmes, Lilongwe, Malawi, 1986.
11. "Potential impact of AIDS on food production and consumption: Tabora case study, Tanzania", unpublished report for FAO.
12. For a study on this in India, see Dogra, B, "The other epidemics" *Economics and Political Weekly*, December 1988, Vol 23, No 50, pp2627-2628, quoted in Corbett, J, "Poverty and sickness: the high cost of ill-health", *IDS Bulletin*, April 1989, Vol 20, No 2, pp58-62.
13. *World Health*, WHO, September/October 1991.
14. Evans, T, "The impact of permanent disability on rural households: river blindness in Guinea", *IDS Bulletin*, April 1989, Vol 20, No 2, pp41-48.
15. Much of the material that follows derives from Barnett, T and Blaikie, P, *AIDS in Africa*, Belhaven Press, London, 1992; and from a report for Panos by Tony Barnett, School of Development Studies, University of East Anglia, UK.
16. Gillespie, S, "Potential impact of AIDS on farming systems: a case study from Rwanda", *Land Use Policy*, 1989, Vol 6, No 4, pp301-312.
17. Ibid.
18. Norse, D, op. cit.
19. Examples taken from Norse, D, op. cit.
20. Ibid.
21. Report for Panos by Tony Barnett, School of Development Studies, University of East Anglia, UK.
22. Abel, N and others, "The impact of AIDS on food production systems in East and Central Africa over the next ten years: a programmatic paper", op. cit.
23. Report for Panos by Tony Barnett, School of Development Studies, University of East Anglia, UK.
24. Arizpe, L, "Relay migration and the survival of the peasant household", in Safa, H I, *Towards a Political Economy of Urbanisation in Third World Countries*, Oxford University Press, New Delhi, 1982, pp20-30.
25. A wide range of credit schemes in Africa, Latin America and Asia are described in *Banking the Unbankable*, Panos, London, 1989.
26. "Responding to AIDS in East Africa: policy and proposals for action", ACORD, 16 June 1992.

CHAPTER 7

1. *African Development Report 1990*, African Development Bank.
2. Interview with Mike Bailey, UNDP, March 1992.
3. *Sunday Times* (South Africa) in *AIDS Newsletter*, 1990/567.
4. *South*, June/July 1991.
5. *Financing and External Debt of Developing Countries: 1990 survey*, OECD, Paris, 1991.
6. *World Development Report 1990*, World Bank.

7. Quote from Unilever representative in report prepared for Panos by Rex Winsburg.
8. Viravaidya, M and others, "The economic impact of AIDS in Thailand", October 1991.
9. Over, M and others, "The direct and indirect cost of HIV infection in developing countries: the cases of Zaire and Tanzania", in Fleming, A and others (eds), *The Global Impact of AIDS*, Alan R Liss Inc, London, 1988.
10. *Human Development Report 1992*, UNDP.
11. Becker, C, "The demo-economic impact of the AIDS pandemic in sub-Saharan Africa", *World Development*, 1990, Vol 18, pp1599-1619.
12. Viravaidya, M and others, op. cit.
13. Shepherd, D S, "Cost of AIDS in a developing area: indirect and direct costs of AIDS in Puerto Rico", in Schwefel, D and others (eds), *Economic Aspects of AIDS and HIV Infection,* Springer, Frankfurt.
14. *Zimbabwe/Malawi Country Report No 2 1992*, Economist Intelligence Unit, London.
15. Ibid.
16. Fraser-Mackenzie, J P, "Commercial Farmers Against AIDS", *AIDS Analysis Africa, Southern Africa Edition*, Vol 2 No 6, 1992.
17. Hore, R, "AIDS and medical aid societies in Zimbabwe", *AIDS Analysis Africa, Southern Africa Edition*, Vol 2, No 4, 1992.
18. *Blaming Others: prejudice, race and worldwide AIDS*, Panos, London, 1988.

CHAPTER 8

1. Interview with Gunilla E rnberg, WHO/GPA, June 1992.
2. Anderson, R and others, "The potential demographic and economic impact of AIDS in sub-Saharan Africa", report to Overseas Development Administration, London, March 1991, p7.
3. For a fuller discussion of this question see *The Third Epidemic: repercussions of the fear of AIDS*, Panos, London, 1990.
4. *The Current Global Situation of the AIDS Pandemic*, WHO Global Progamme on AIDS, Geneva, July 1992.
5. See, for example, *Abstracts of VIth International Conference on AIDS in Africa*, Dakar, 1991, MO 126, MO 127 and MA 153.
6. *AIDS Analysis Africa*, July/August 1991.
7. Presentation by Michael Helquist, VIth International Conference on AIDS, San Francisco, June 1990.
8. Information from Health Education Authority, London, September 1992.
9. See, for example, Baitwababo, C, "Living positively as a peer educator", *Abstracts of VIIIth International Conference on AIDS*, Amsterdam, 1992, PuD 9013.
10. Points taken from interview with Gary Slutkin, Global Programme on AIDS, WHO, June 1992.
11. *National Mirror*, Lusaka, 6 April 1991.
12. Information from Veriano Terto Jr, ABIA, July 1992.
13. Wilson, D and others, "Prevention du SIDA auprès de lycéens en Afrique de L'Ouest: l'experience d'un concours d'information", *Abstracts of VIth International Conference on AIDS in Africa*, Dakar, 1991, MA 152.
14. Williams, E and others, "Nigeria: empowering commercial sex workers for HIV prevention", *Abstracts of VIIth International Conference on AIDS*, Florence, 1991, WD 4041.

15. WHO Press Release WHO/44, 22 June 1992.

16. Ibid.

17. Costa, N and others, "Integrated strategies targeting female sex workers and clients in Rio de Janeiro", poster presentation, VIIIth International Conference on AIDS, Amsterdam, 1992.

18. Thanprasertsuk, S and others, *Thai AIDS Journal*, 1991, Vol 3, pp54-60, in *AIDS Newsletter*, 1992/360.

19. Personal communication, 26 August 1992.

20. Address to VIth International Conference on AIDS in Africa, Dakar, December 1991.

21. Interview with Susan Foster, December 1991; Ndeki, S and others, "AIDS knowledge and risk behaviour among primary school children in Arusha and Kagera regions, Tanzania", *Abstracts of VIIIth International Conference on AIDS*, Amsterdam, 1992, PuD 9129.

22. Interview with Mike Bailey, UNDP, February 1992.

23. Many studies support this: see, for example, Allen, S and others, "Effect of serotesting with counselling on condom use and seroconversion among HIV discordant couples in Africa", *British Medical Journal*, 1992, Vol 304, pp1605-1609.

24. Quote and examples from Liskin, L, "Progress for developing countries", *AIDS Care*, 1989, Vol 1, No 2, pp199-202.

25. Address to VIth International Conference on AIDS in Africa, Dakar, December 1991.

26. Interview, May 1992.

27. Interview, February 1992.

28. *Africa Health*, September 1991.

29. Point derived from Elias C, "Sexually transmitted diseases and the reproductive health of women in developing countries", *Population Council Programs Division Working Paper 5*, 1991.

30. Grant, R and others, "Trends of HIV seroprevalence and risk behaviors in STD patients in Uganda", *Abstracts of VIIIth International Conference on AIDS*, Amsterdam, 1992, PoC 4022.

31. Interview with Sue Lucas, May 1992.

32. Population Services International, Washington, September 1992.

33. *Financial Gazette*, Harare, 30 November 1990.

34. Whiteside, A, "HIV infection and AIDS in Zimbabwe: an assessment", South African Foundation for Economic Research, Harare, 1991.

35. Correspondence with Steven Forsythe, health finance research associate at Family Health International, June 1992.

36. Ibid.

37. Ibid.

38. Based on Over, M and others, "The direct and indirect cost of HIV infection in developing countries: the cases of Zaire and Tanzania", *The Global Impact of AIDS*, Allan R Liss Inc, New York, 1988.

39. Moses, S and others, "Controlling HIV in Africa: effectiveness and cost of intervention in a high-frequency STD transmitter core group", *AIDS*, 1991, Vol 5, pp407-411.

40. Standaert, B and Comité Scientifique du Sida au Burundi, "Economic and social determinants on the AIDS epidemic in Burundi" in Giraldi, G and others (eds), *AIDS and Associated Cancers in Africa*, Basel, 1988. For further discussion of the cost benefits of preventing further cases of HIV/AIDS, see Bertozzi, S,

"Combating HIV in Africa: a role for economic research", *AIDS*, 1991, Vol 5, ppS45-S54; and Over, M and Piot, P, "HIV infection and other sexually transmitted diseases", in Jamison, D and Mosley, W (eds), *Evolving Health Sector Priorities in Developing Countries*, World Bank, forthcoming.

41. Viravaidya, M and others, "Economic impact of AIDS on Thailand", October 1991.

42. Tarantola, D and others, "How much is spent on AIDS in the world and where does the money go?", paper presented at VIIIth International Conference on AIDS, Amsterdam, 1992.

43. Ibid.

44. Anderson, R and others, op. cit., pp8-9

45. N'Galy, B and others, "Obstacles to the optimal management of HIV infection/AIDS in Africa", *Journal of Acquired Immune Deficiency Syndromes*, 1990, Vol 3, pp430-437.

46. Ibid.

47. N'tita, I and others, "Risk of transfusion-associated HIV transmission in Kinshasa, Zaire", *AIDS*, 1991, Vol 5, pp437-439.

48. De Moya, E A and others, "The Costs and Benefits of HIV Blood Donor Screening Systems in Trinidad and Tobago, The Dominican Republic and the Philippines", Family Health International, US, June 1992.

49. Panos guesstimate extrapolated from estimates of injecting drug use population in the United States and Europe given by Coutinho, R, "Epidemiology and prevention of AIDS among intravenous drug users", *Journal of Acquired Immune Deficiency Syndromes*, 1990, Vol 3, pp413-416.

50. WHO Press Release, WHO/44, 22 June 1992.

51. *Abstracts of VIth International Conference on AIDS in Africa*, Dakar, 1991, TO 131-TO 137; WA 228-WA 249.

52. *AIDS Analysis Africa*, July/August 1991.

53. Gangakhedkar, R and Apte, S, "Barriers in condom acceptance in a rural population of India", *Abstracts of VIIIth International Conference on AIDS*, Amsterdam, 1992, PuC 8082.

54. Munyakho, D, "Rural realities and condom use", *WorldAIDS*, May 1991, No 15, Panos, London.

CHAPTER 9

1. Panos estimate.

2. "Financial Information on 1991 Income and Obligations", WHO document GPA/GMC(8)/92.8 Rev 1, 9 June 1992.

3. *New Scientist*, London, 1 February 1992.

4. *AIDS Analysis Africa*, July/August 1991.

5. "WHO/UNDP Alliance to combat AIDS", GPA/ER/88.1.

6. Interview, May 1992; letter, August 1992.

7. Interview, August 1992.

8. Interview, January 1991.

9. *AIDS Analysis Africa*, November/December 1991.

10. Address given at VIth International Conference on AIDS in Africa, Dakar, December 1991.

11. Merson, M, "AIDS in the 1990s: meeting the challenge", paper presented at annual World Bank/IMF meeting, Bangkok, Thailand, October 1991.

12. "Responding to AIDS in East Africa: policy and proposals for action", ACORD, June 1992.